TRACE ELEMENTS and OTHER ESSENTIAL NUTRIENTS

Clinical Application of Tissue Mineral Analysis

by
Dr. David L. Watts

TRACE ELEMENTS AND OTHER ESSENTIAL NUTRIENTS. Copyright © 1995 by Dr. David L. Watts. All rights reserved. Printed in the United States of America. No part of this book may be used or reproduced in any manner whatsoever without written permission except in the case of brief quotations embodied in critical articles and reviews. For information address Trace Elements, 4901 Keller Springs Road, Dallas, Texas 75248.

2nd Writer's B-L-O-C-K- edition published 1997

Watts, David L.
    Trace elements and other essential nutrients.

    "Writer's B-L-O-C-K-"
    1. Endocrinology 2. Nutrition 3. Health 4. Fitness I. Title. II. Subtitle

Library of Congress Catalog Card Number 95-079696
ISBN 1-885676-15-8

Dedication

This book is dedicated to my parents, Herbert and Evelyn, for their encouragement; to my wife Barbara, for her unending support; and to Tim for his motivation. I also want to thank Beth Ellyn for her enthusiastic insights.

Introduction

The understanding of nutrition and its important role in health is continually developing and gaining prominence. Nutrition is becoming more accepted as an intricate part of health care, particularly among today's progressive health care professionals.

Nutrition no longer deals simply with single nutrient deficiencies, but with disturbed metabolic functions, nutrient imbalances, and prevention of chronic and degenerative disease. It is estimated by researchers that diet is involved in over thirty percent of cancers, and over forty percent of heart disease, the two major causes of death in the United States.

However, new discoveries in nutritional knowledge is often slow to be accepted among the so-called scientific community, both past and present. It took years for the acceptance that scurvy could be prevented by the consumption of citrus. Oftentimes, crew members of ships carrying limes to the British Navy succumbed to the effects of scurvy even though they possessed a shipload of prevention. It took over 30 years before the widespread acceptance that beriberi was caused by a vitamin B deficiency rather than a bacteria. Only a couple of decades ago the American Medical establishment stated unequivocally that diet had no effect upon the incidence of cancer, but now the American Cancer Society sends out information material to the public emphasizing that diet does indeed help to prevent many forms of cancer.

The problem is that there is a great deal of confusion in the field of nutrition. Records of food intake in groups with chronic disease look generally the same as those of a healthy population. Part, if not most of this confusion, is due to the failure to recognize that there is a major difference between diet and nutrition which should be distinguished. Diet consists of what is consumed, whereas nutrition, which is more important, is what is obtained from the foods and further, what is excreted unused. Nutrition, especially as it pertains to trace elements, involves more than just consuming foods from the basic food groups. There are many factors that affect nutrient utilization such as:

1) Individual metabolic characteristics; 2) Neurological activity; 3) Endocrine function; 4) Bioavailability of nutrients in foods; 5) Specific dynamic action of foods; 6) Absorption at the intestinal level; 7) Utilization at the cellular level; 8) Synergism and antagonism between minerals and vitamins; 9) Environmental pollutants, or xenobiotics; and 10) Stress. Even our emotional status affects nutritional requirements. Awareness and understanding of these factors is the major difference between the nutritional-oriented doctor, or health care professional, and dietetics. Dietetics involve preparing a well-rounded diet, or specialized diets for patients with specific diseases. Nutritionists on the other hand, are more concerned with the nutritional biochemistry of the individual. Health of the human body as a whole begins at the cellular level. Whether nutrients are reaching the cellular level, and what the consequence are of too much or too little, is the major concern of nutritionists today.

Only recently has the role of trace elements been appreciated. Mineral deficiencies and imbalances are known to affect and be involved in disorders of the cardiovascular system, gastrointestinal, muscular, skeletal, neurological, immune and endocrine systems. This has lead to even more confusion, since minerals are interrelated with each other, as well as being linked with the metabolism of proteins, carbohydrates, fats, and of course, vitamins.

The development of tissue mineral analysis (TMA) of human hair through atomic spectroscopy techniques and the proper interpretation of these results has helped considerably in understanding the complex relationship of minerals in the body. Hair is an easily obtained biopsy material of the body. Within this biopsy material is contained the minerals incorporated during its development. Multiple minerals can be tested and the mineral interrelationships of the body are displayed. This information represents not only the nutritional status of the individual, but reflects the neuroendocrine activity as well. With proper interpretation, an individual's metabolic activity and the complex nutrient interrelationships within the body can be screened.

With this wealth of information available to us today, we can no longer take lightly the role of nutrition in health and disease. Nutritional recommendations should not be based simply on external symptoms, the latest fad, or a "shotgun" approach. In fact, the nutritional treatment of an individual, or the correction of metabolic disturbances, should be directed toward bringing the entire metabolic environment into a more ideal balance.

Table of Contents

1 DETERMINING NUTRITIONAL STATUS FROM HAIR TISSUE MINERAL ANALYSIS — 1

Assessment Of Mineral Status 2
How Is A Hair Sample Analyzed? 5
What About Contamination Of The Hair? 6
How Can TMA Indicate Vitamin Needs? 7
Advantages Of Hair TMA 8
Interpretation Of TMA Results 9

2 NUTRITIONAL RELATIONSHIPS — 15

Synergistic And Antagonistic Relationships 15
Mineral Interrelationships - Antagonism 16
Mineral Synergism 17
Vitamin Interrelationships - Antagonism 18
Vitamin Synergism 19
Vitamin-Mineral Interrelationships - Antagonism 20
Vitamin-Mineral Synergism 21

3 NUTRITIONAL-ENDOCRINE RELATIONSHIPS — 24

Sympathetic And Parasympathetic Nervous System 24
The Endocrine Glands 25
Nutritional Effects Of The Neuro-Endocrine System 27
Factors Affecting Endocrine Activity 28
Nutrients Involved In The Alarm Stage Of Stress 29
Nutrients Involved In The Resistance Stage Of Stress 29
Nutrients Required In The Recovery Stage Of Stress 29

4 METABOLIC INDIVIDUALITY — 33

Tissue Mineral Analysis And Metabolic Types 34
The Fast Metabolizer 35
Factors Contributing To Fast Metabolism 36
Slow Metabolism 37
Factors Contributing To A Slow Metabolic Rate 38
Advantage Of Knowing One's Metabolic Type 41
Classification Of Disease Processes 41

Conditions Associated With Sympathetic Dominance 42
Conditions Associated With Para-sympathetic Dominance 42
Classification Of Nutrients - Vitamins And Minerals 42
Water 43
Foods 44
Herbs 48
Drugs 49

5 CALCIUM   52

Calcium Regulation 53
Osteoporosis 54
Type I Osteoporosis 56
Type II Osteoporosis 57
Factors Associated With Too Little Tissue Calcium 58
Calcium Supplements And Depression 59
Other Factors Associated With Too Much Tissue Calcium 60
Blood Calcium 61
Hypocalcemia 61
Hypercalcemia 62
Vitamin-Mineral Synergists 62

6 MAGNESIUM   66

Problems Created By Magnesium Deficiencies 67
Increased Perspiration And Body Odor 67
Muscle Cramps 67
Cardio-Vascular Conditions 68
Arthritis-Stones-Bursitis 69
Urinary Frequency - Constipation 69
Toxic Shock Syndrome 69
Insomnia 70
Epilepsy-Seizure Disorders-Pregnancy 70
Causes Of Magnesium Deficiencies 70
The Endocrine Glands And Magnesium 71
Minerals Antagonistic To Magnesium 72
Vitamins Antagonistic To Magnesium 74
Vitamin-Mineral Synergists 75

7 COPPER   78

Conditions Associated With Copper Deficiency 78
Copper And Anemia 79
Copper And Arthritis 79
Bacterial Infections 80
Neurological Disorders 81
Cardiovascular Disorders 82
Malignancies And Copper 82

Conditions Associated With Copper Toxicity 83
Premenstrual Syndrome (PMS) And Copper 84
Toxemia And Post Partum Depression 85
Gallstones 85
Viral And Bacterial Infections 86
Yeast And Fungus 87
Scoliosis 87
Copper And Mental Function 88
Medications That May Contribute To Copper Toxicity 90
Endocrine Effects Upon Copper 90
Copper And The Thyroid 90
Copper And The Adrenal Glands 91
Factors Contributing To Copper Deficiency: Minerals 91
Vitamins 92
Synergistic Nutrients 93

8 ZINC 96

Zinc Deficiency 96
Skin Conditions 97
Nails 98
Sickle Cell Anemia 98
Diabetes 98
Anorexia Nervosa 98
Menstrual Irregularities 99
Viruses 99
Why A Zinc Deficiency Develops 100
Zinc Overload 100
Minerals And Vitamins Antagonistic To Zinc 101
Synergistic Nutrients 103
Tissue Mineral Analysis (TMA) And Zinc Analysis 103
Zinc Requirements 103

9 IRON 106

Mental Effects Of Iron 107
Other Conditions Associated With Iron Imbalance 107
Pica 108
Dysphagia 108
Iron And Infections 109
Iron Overload 109
The Endocrine (Hormonal) Effects Of Iron Imbalance 111
Minerals Antagonistic To Iron 112
Vitamins Antagonistic To Iron 113
Iron Requirements 114

10 MANGANESE — 117

- How Your Body Utilizes Manganese 118
- Hormonal Effects Upon Manganese 118
- Manganese And Diet 118
- Manganese Deficiency 119
- Manganese Toxicity 121

11 CHROMIUM — 124

- Chromium Deficiency-Diabetes 124
- Peripheral Neuropathy 125
- Cardiovascular Heart Disease (CHD) 125
- Hormonal Factors Contributing to Chromium Deficiency -Insulin 125
- Estrogen 126
- Thyroid, Para-Thyroid 126
- Stress 126
- Factors Contributing To Chromium Deficiency - Dietary 127
- Minerals 127
- Chromium Requirements 129

12 SELENIUM — 132

- Selenium Toxicity And Deficiency In Animals 133
- Selenium In Human Nutrition - Deficiency 134
- Cataracts 134
- Red Blood Cell (Erythrocyte) Disorders 135
- Aging 135
- Cancer 135
- Immune Competence 136
- Sudden Infant Death Syndrome (SIDS) 136
- Cystic Fibrosis 136
- Crohn's Disease 136
- Thyroid 137
- Factors Contributing To Selenium Deficiency 137
- Nutrients Synergistic To Selenium 139
- Human Selenium Toxicity 140
- Sources Of Selenium 140
- Symptoms Of Selenium Toxicity 140
- Sources Of Selenium And Body Distribution 141
- Assessment Of Selenium Status 142

13 SODIUM, POTASSIUM, CHLORIDE   147

Requirements 147
Regulation 148
Deficiency 149
Excesses 150
Hypertension 150
Factors Contributing To Sodium Chloride Sensitivity 151
Sodium, Potassium And TMA Studies 153

14 TOXIC AND OTHER METALS   156

Lead (Pb) 157
Arsenic (As) 159
Beryllium (Be) 160
Cadmium (Cd) 160
Mercury (Hg) 161
Aluminum (Al) 162

Ultra Trace Elements 162
Antimony (Sb) 162
Barium (Ba) 163
Boron (B) 163
Cobalt (Co) 163
Germanium (Ge) 165
Gold (Au) 165
Lithium (Li) 165
Molybdenum (Mo) 166
Nickel (Ni) 167
Platinum (Pt) 168
Silicon (Si) 168
Strontium (Sr) 169
Sulfur (S) 169
Silver (Ag) 169
Tin (Sn) 170
Titanium (Ti) 170
Vanadium (V) 170
Zirconium (Zr) 171

INDEX   176

Chapter 1

Determining Nutritional Status From Hair Tissue Mineral Analysis

Minerals comprise approximately four percent of our total body weight and include macro and micro elements. The macroelements are those found in the body in high concentrations, such as calcium, phosphorus, sodium, potassium, and sulfur. Microelements, or trace elements, are present in low concentrations and include elements such as chromium, vanadium, selenium, lithium and manganese. Their functions range from providing structural support in the formation of bones and teeth, to maintaining the acid-base balance, water balance, nerve conduction, muscle contraction, and enzyme functions. Some minerals participate in hundreds of biochemical processes, while others participate in only limited functions. Their role in health and disease is just recently being recognized, such as their involvement in the prevention of cancer, immune regulation, chronic degenerative diseases, aging, and even emotions. In the words of the late Dr. Henry Schroeder, "Minerals are the basic spark-plugs in the chemistry of life, on which the exchanges of energy in the combustion of foods and the building of living tissues depend." This statement emphasizes the extreme importance of essential minerals in biological systems for optimum function and health.

Even though the essential minerals are necessary in adequate amounts for health, excessive accumulation can also prove detrimental. Two examples are iron and copper. Iron can accumulate in the body to the point of toxicity, known as hemochromatosis, or hemosiderosis. Too much copper accumulation can cause liver degeneration and brain disorders known as hepatolenticular degeneration, or more commonly, Wilson's Disease. The presence of an imbalance between these minerals is also known to contribute to health problems, therefore their balance within the body is proving just as important as their individual levels.

Other minerals that are also present in the body have little or no beneficial effects. These are the heavy metals such as lead, cadmium and mercury. They are called heavy metals due to their high atomic weight, which allow them to displace many of the lighter, essential elements, and are considered toxic. Heavy metals are ever present in our environment, therefore, they are also found to some extent in all biological systems.

Assessment Of Mineral Status

Assessment of the essential and non-essential elements is very important not only for determining adequacy and deficiencies, but also for assessing their relative relationships. A test has been developed that serves this purpose exceedingly well. This test is known as tissue mineral analysis, or TMA. The most common tissue used for this purpose is hair. As the hair is being formed, prior to extrusion from the scalp, it is exposed to the blood, lymph, and intracellular fluids. During this time, it accumulates constituents present in this internal environment, particularly the minerals, but other substances as well. As the cortex of the hair shaft hardens and protrudes from the scalp, the evidence of this internal metabolic environment is preserved as a convenient record. Even drugs consumed during this developmental process will be present.

Human hair has been accepted as an effective tissue for biological monitoring of toxic heavy metals by the U.S. Environmental Protection Agency, and is being used for this purpose throughout the world. It is ideal in that it fits the following criteria: 1) Hair accumulates all the important trace elements; 2) It is a commonly available tissue; 3) It is widespread geographically; 4) Hair is easily collected, stored and transported; 5) It is suitable since specimens can be resampled; 6) It is present in polluted and non-polluted areas; 7) The content of the hair correlates with environmental gradients of metals; 8) There is sufficient background and exposure data making hair especially suitable for biological monitoring for exposure assessment as well as global, regional, and local surveillance monitoring; and 9) The use of hair has advantages over other tissues. Monitoring metals in the urine measures the component that is absorbed, but excreted. The blood measures the component that is absorbed and temporarily in circulation before it is excreted and/or sequestered into storage depots.

Hair analysis studies have shown it to be an excellent tissue to monitor toxic metal exposure in humans and animals. For example, animals receiving 300 parts per million of cadmium in drinking water had an average intake of 4.5 milligrams over 12 weeks. Peak levels were reached in the liver, kidneys and hair in 4 weeks. In animals exposed to lesser amounts, a peak was reached at 7 weeks in the kidneys, and 9 weeks in the liver and hair. Blood levels during this time remained consistently low despite continuous exposure and did not correlate with kidney or liver concentrations. However, the hair cadmium levels did correlate with kidney and liver concentrations. It has been concluded by this and many other studies that hair can be used as an indicator of whole-body accumulation, and that blood is not a good indicator of accumulation.

Hair and blood analyses were performed in a nation-wide survey of children living near smelters. These were compared to children not living near smelters. Over 1,000 children were included in the study, ranging from 1-5 years of age. Blood levels of heavy metals were not elevated in most of the exposed children. However, elevated hair levels of lead and cadmium were detected and provided evidence of exposure that should be reduced.

A study of individuals suffering from mercury-induced kidney disease found hair to be the most useful tissue in determining mercury toxicity. Patients were exposed to mercury through the use of skin lightening creams. The mercury was absorbed through the skin and resulted in the nephrotic syndrome. Mercury levels in the hair have also been related to the frequency of fish consumption. Studies have included hair testing of hundreds of individuals in over 13 countries. The results of the study correlated the mercury found in the hair with mercury ingested from contaminated seafood.

Hair has been used for many years as an indicator for nutritional status and nutritional supplementation in animals. Hundreds of studies have correlated the levels of minerals in feed and hair of cattle. Hair is used to monitor nutritional status of animals related to fertility and disease, and hair manganese levels have been correlated with hydroxyproline levels (a manganese activated enzyme) in mice. Hair copper has shown a correlation with liver concentrations in animals which indicates its use to assess nutritional status in man. Nutritional assessment in humans has also been common. Dr. A. Prasad is well known for his studies of zinc deficiency in patients suffering from dwarfism. He found low hair zinc levels in those affected. Supplementing zinc resulted in increased production of growth hormones that contributed to increased growth and development in the affected group. The hair zinc levels were found to increase as well. Low hair zinc levels have been found in children with failure to thrive, and slow growth rates. Zinc supplementation resulted in increased growth rates, elevated growth hormones, and increased hair zinc levels. Hair analysis has been extremely useful in detecting nutritional disturbances in many disease states. The most recognized are cystic fibrosis, acrodermatitis enteropathica, cirrhosis, sickle cell disease, PKU, Kaschin-Beck and Keshan Disease, cardiovascular disease, diabetes, mental disturbances, and many others.

Hair analysis can also be used to evaluate the nutritional status and toxic metal exposure of the fetus through testing the mother's hair, as well as monitoring the use of prescribed and illicit drugs.

Hair TMAs have been performed for over 30 years. Therefore, laboratory procedures and techniques are now well established. Even with this wealth of experience, TMA is still criticized and questioned as to its validity. Most, if not all, of the criticism directed toward hair mineral analysis is from data that is over 20 years old. However, there has been a great deal of research over the past 25 years, leading to improved laboratory techniques and procedures. Testing instruments are far advanced over the early equipment. Advances in this area can be compared to the advancements in computer technology, which everyone knows is never at a standstill. Over the past few decades, virtually millions of analytical tests have been performed on hair samples obtained from individuals throughout the world. Laboratory techniques, procedures, instrumentation, and reporting have been well refined. In fact, it should be noted that all laboratories which provide TMA testing are licensed and certified by state and federal regulatory agencies. When a hair sample is properly obtained, analyzed and interpreted, it has proven to be an economical screening tool for toxic metal exposure as well as a good indicator of nutrient interrelationships and nutritional status. Routine hair mineral analysis is an excellent tool to complement other clinical tests.

In the past, much of this criticism was warranted, but much mis-information and hearsay were also put forth. The most common questions concerning TMA will be discussed in the following sections.

How Is A Hair Sample Analyzed?

The hair should be taken from the scalp at several different locations. These areas include the sub-occipital region, or nape of the neck, to the mid vertex, or very top of the head, and temporal regions. The hair should be cut at the scalp and only the proximal one and one-half inches should be used for analysis. Sample weight requirements vary from lab to lab depending upon the analytical technique used, usually from 200 milligrams to as much as one gram of hair. In addition, each lab often requests that slightly more sample weight be submitted, so that confirmatory rechecks can be performed when found to be necessary.

Once the sample arrives in most laboratories, it will normally undergo four phases of processing involving: login; preparation and digestion; analysis; and report processing. The login phase involves the assignment of an identification number and entry into the report processing and billing systems. The preparation and digestion phase involves the careful cutting and weighing of the sample. This phase also includes the use of multiple acids and high temperature to break down the structure of the hair. Once the digestion is completed, only the mineral components of the hair in the form of mineral salts remain. At this point, the sample is rehydrated with a reagent solution to put the minerals into suspension. The sample is then ready for analysis. The analysis phase involves the use of highly sophisticated equipment and techniques, of which the most common are atomic absorption spectroscopy and plasma emission spectroscopy. Whichever technique is used, the sample is aspirated into the instrument where each mineral is then measured. The units of measurement for reporting test results will vary from lab to lab, but will be in either milligrams percent (mg%) or parts-per-million (ppm). Each of the above three phases, particularly the preparation and analytical phases, are controlled by very strict laboratory procedures and reporting protocol. These standards help to insure both accuracy and precision on a daily basis. The final phase, which is report processing, involves the transfer of test data to a computer processing system. This system uses sophisticated programs that interpret the test data and create customized reports. Additionally, the system also prints graphs which graphically display the individual test results as compared to that laboratory's established reference ranges and normals. An example of a TMA graph is shown in two parts, figures 1a and 1b.

What About Contamination Of The Hair?

It is critically important to be aware of the possible contaminants that can affect laboratory results of any biological sample. The use of iron scissors that have developed rust when cutting a hair sample can result in artificially elevated iron. The use of cracked or peeling chrome plated instruments can also present a potential problem, contributing to chromium contamination. Therefore, only high grade stainless steel instruments should be used to cut the hair sample.

Dyes that blacken the hair typically contain lead acetate, which contributes to excessively high lead levels in the hair. A sample obtained from someone using such a product can be considered unreliable for determining lead status. If the laboratory finds an exorbitant amount of lead in the test result, the lab report will indicate the possibility of a contamination. If the patient is in fact using a hair dye, then it would be suggested that other body hair be submitted for lead determination. Pubic, axillary, or chest hair can be used for this purpose, since it is usually unexposed to the dye. If other body hair is not available, nails may be used. Lead contamination from such dyes do not adversely affect the rest of the mineral results. It should be pointed out that lead contained in various cosmetic preparations can be absorbed through the skin, and thereby contribute to body burdens of this heavy metal. This has prompted some countries to ban lead containing products of this type.

Anti-dandruff, or medicated shampoos, can contribute to excessive selenium results, and bleaching of the hair will add to the calcium findings. Permanent wave solutions contain magnesium and can artificially elevate magnesium findings. Most clinical laboratories are very aware of contaminants in various hair preparations. The best samples to submit for testing are ones that have not been treated, or, one can wait for the hair to grow sufficiently so that only untreated hair can be obtained. It should be noted that these contaminants appear to affect only the individual mineral contaminant, and not the other minerals tested.

This often brings up the question regarding environmental contamination of samples. For instance, if a person lives near a lead smelter, will the industrial release settle on the surface of the hair? This certainly can be the case. However, if this occurs, one should be aware that the entire body is also being exposed. Internal accumulation occurs through the lungs, by absorption through the skin, as well as absorption from the digestive tract, due to eating foods that have been exposed. So hair is an excellent media for determining environmental exposure.

Often people ask if pubic hair should be the primary source for analysis since it is not usually treated. The growth rate and physiology of other body hair is different from scalp hair. Therefore, scalp samples are always more preferable than any other type of sample. Samples from pubic, axillary, and chest should only be used for confirmation purposes. Of course this is not always possible, so if a scalp sample is absolutely not available, then other body hair can be used. If there is no body hair available, then nail samples can be used as the third choice.

How Can TMA Indicate Vitamin Needs?

This is probably the next most frequent question and is also frequently used as one of its criticisms. If hair is used to test for minerals, how can it be used to determine vitamin needs, since vitamins are not found in the hair? This is not such a mystery when one understands the relationship of vitamins to minerals. For example, if a patient is suffering from rickets, which is a calcium metabolism disturbance, vitamin D is usually the first recommendation. This is usually done without ever testing for vitamin D status. Therefore, if a very low calcium level is found on a TMA result, it would be safe to say that not only calcium is needed, but chances are there is also an increased vitamin D requirement. Zinc metabolism needs adequate amounts of vitamin B_6. Copper relates to vitamin C requirements, and vitamin C is known to aid iron absorption. The activity of vitamin A is greatly impaired during zinc deficiency. So the status of a mineral can give a strong indication of a vitamin need, especially when vitamin-mineral synergisms and antagonisms are taken into consideration.

Advantages Of Hair TMA

Tissue mineral analysis (TMA) of the hair offers a number of advantages in helping to determine mineral needs. First, since the hair is a fairly slow growing tissue, there are no daily fluctuations. For instance, if you eat bananas before having a blood test taken, your blood potassium level may be high that day. If you have your blood tested the next day and did not eat bananas, your blood potassium may be normal, or even low. The TMA potassium level will be reflective of overall, or long term dietary habits rather than what is consumed just for a day or two. Furthermore, TMA reflects the storage levels of minerals rather than just what is being transported in the blood. Trace element concentrations of the hair represents time-weighted exposure values which make it more useful for epidemiological and nutritional studies. Hair testing is also well suited for environmental and forensic investigations.

Another advantage is that many minerals can be tested with only one properly obtained sample. These include toxic heavy metals such as lead, mercury, cadmium, and aluminum. This makes TMA one of the most extensive, as well as economical screening tools available today.

Hair mineral levels have to be interpreted carefully as well. For example, a normal hair zinc level does not necessarily indicate an adequate level. However, a low level in the hair strongly indicates a potential deficiency. The most important contribution of TMA is not in determining absolute deficiencies, but rather its ability to reveal relative imbalances between nutrients. It is one of the best aids we have in the field of nutrition that provides information for balancing body chemistry. In today's modern societies, we are finding that imbalances between nutrients are much more common than deficiencies of individual nutrients.

TMA also provides another avenue for the exploration of an individual's health status. For example, if a patient presents symptoms and the cause cannot be determined through other tests, a TMA can direct the clinician toward a specific area of the chemistry that may be involved. If the TMA is used as the primary, or first clinical test, it can indicate other laboratory tests to support the findings.

Recently, a doctor sent a sample to our laboratory from a patient that had undergone extensive blood tests costing several thousand dollars. She was suffering from a myriad of symptoms, fatigue being one of the most prevalent. All previous tests were negative and revealed no abnormalities. The patient's previous doctor told her that all the tests would have to be repeated. Instead, she decided to see another doctor who submitted her hair sample for analysis. The patient began following the recommendations based upon the TMA. Within six weeks, the patient markedly improved. This emphasizes the importance of treating the patient instead of the symptom. We found an imbalance in the patient's chemistry through the TMA and addressed it.

Another example involves an infant. Shortly after birth, the child developed a number of symptoms including seizures and irritability. The child was twitching and moving constantly when awake. The child's physical development was severely retarded. Extensive work-ups and examinations by a well known hospital provided little information as to what was contributing to these problems. After many months with no significant improvement, the mother asked another doctor about a nutritional approach. A hair TMA was then performed. After reviewing the TMA results, we found significant imbalances in the child's profile. Therapy was suggested based upon the TMA. Two months later it was reported that the child was markedly improving. The child had gained weight and the seizures had improved to the point that the seizure medication, phenobarbital, was discontinued.

Interpretation Of TMA Results

The results from any laboratory test have little value unless they are interpreted properly. For example, what would be the significance of an elevated alkaline phosphatase (an enzyme in the serum) if found in a person's blood test? With only this much information there is not much that could be concluded. However, if we know the test was done on a child, elevation of this particular enzyme may be perfectly normal. If the test was from an individual who had recently broken some bones, elevation of this enzyme would also be normal. Other factors that can affect this enzyme include strenuous exercise, pregnancy, and chronic alcoholism. Medications may also cause an elevation of the enzyme. However, some disease process are specifically related to increased levels of the enzyme such as pancreatitis, liver and bone disease, and hyperthyroidism. Other blood tests would have to be done to help confirm the reason for an elevation of the enzyme. The history of the patient would also have to be obtained. In other words, all of this information would have to be considered when interpreting the significance of this one enzyme.

The same care and scrutiny must be applied when interpreting the results of TMA patterns. For example, just looking at a tissue zinc level means very little. Zinc must be evaluated with other significant factors for the results to be useful. Meaningful information cannot be determined unless the zinc results are related, and/or compared to its co-factors, such as the individual's metabolic type, calcium, copper and iron status. Potassium levels and the sodium to potassium relationship as well as the calcium to potassium relationship, also help in evaluating the significance of zinc, as well as zinc's relationship to heavy metals such as mercury, cadmium, and lead. Calcium, for instance, must be evaluated not only by the level found on the TMA result, but in conjunction with phosphorus, magnesium, sodium, potassium, and lead, as well as the age and sex of the individual being tested.

At Trace Elements, a specially designed computer program helps in the interpretation of TMA results. This highly sophisticated program is constantly being updated according to the latest research performed at our laboratory as well as from research information obtained from universities and institutes throughout the world. When an individual's test results are entered into the computer, literally thousands of computations and comparisons are made in order to interpret the results properly. The computations range from evaluating the metabolic type, to comparison of mineral levels and ratios, to evaluating the relationship of heavy metals to nutrient mineral levels. Endocrine assessments are made based upon the factors that are known to affect or control mineral metabolism. Even dietary factors are related to the mineral patterns. This includes the levels and ratios of minerals in foods, water and herbs, in relation to the individual laboratory results.

The clinician can then use this information in conjunction with the patient's other clinical tests, history, and health condition in designing a specific and individualized approach to therapy.

Conclusion

A hair sample, when properly obtained, analyzed, and interpreted, can provide specific information about one's metabolic and nutritional status. This includes the effects of diet, nutritional supplementation, stress, toxic metal exposure, and even inherited mineral patterns.

Through clinical results and continuing research, TMA is gaining a wide reputation internationally. It is being utilized as an effective screening tool in conjunction with other diagnostic tests by physicians, nutritionists, and other health care providers in many countries. Hair is one of the most readily accessible tissues to examine, and given the vast amount of information a TMA can yield, it is one of the most economical nutritional tests available today.

The following is a list of the thirty-six minerals routinely tested at Trace Elements, Inc.

NUTRITIONAL MINERALS				
Calcium	Magnesium	Sodium	Potassium	Copper
Zinc	Phosphorus	Iron	Manganese	Chromium
Selenium	Boron	Cobalt	Germanium	Molybdenum
Silicon	Sulfur	Vanadium	Antimony	Barium
Silver	Lithium	Nickel	Platinum	Gold
Strontium	Tin	Titanium	Tungsten	Zirconium
HEAVY METALS				
Arsenic	Beryllium	Mercury	Cadmium	Lead
Aluminum				

TRACE ELEMENTS and OTHER ESSENTIAL NUTRIENTS

Figure 1a
Graph Of Hair TMA

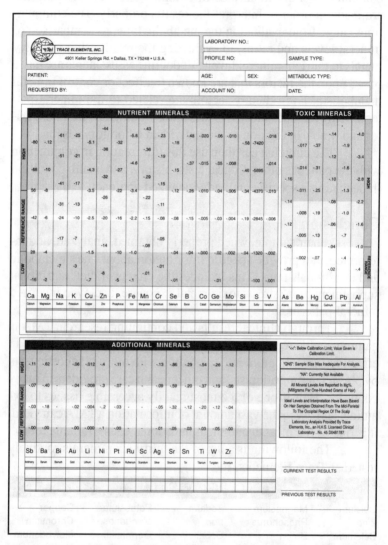

Figure 1b
Graph Of Hair TMA

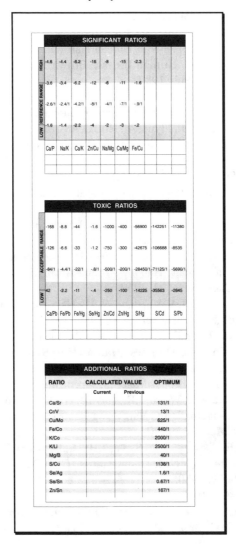

References

Hopps, H.C: The Biological Bases for Using Hair and Nail for Analysis of Trace Elements. **Sci.Tot.Environ.** 7, 1977.

Gilbert, R.I: Trace Elements in Human Hair and Bone. **Hair, Trace Elements and Human Illness.** Brown, A.C., Crounse, R.G., Eds. Praeger Pub. 1980.

Rybukhin, T.S: International Coordinated Program on Activation Analysis of Trace Element Pollutants in Human Hair. **Ibid.**

Strain, W.H., Pories, W.J., Flynn, A., Hill, O.A: Trace Element Nutriture and Metabolism Through Head Hair Analysis. **Trace Substances in Environmental Health.** Hemphill, D., Ed. Univ. Mo. Press, Columbia. 1972.

Katz, S.A: The Use of Hair As a Biopsy Material for Trace Elements in the Body. **Am.Lab.** Feb., 1979.

Laker, M: On Determining Trace Element Levels in Man: The Uses of Blood and Hair. **Lancet** 11, 1982.

Harrison, W., Yurchek, J., Benson, C: The Determination of Trace Elements in Human Hair by Atomic Absorption Spectroscopy. **Clin.Chem.Acta.** 23, 1969.

Baumgartner, W.A., Hill, V.A., Blahd, W.H: Hair Analysis for Drugs of Abuse. **J.Forensic Sci.** 34, 6, 1989.

Kopito, L., Shwachman, H: Alterations in the Elemental Composition of Hair in Some Diseases. **Human Hair Symposium.** Brown, A., Ed. Medicon Press, N.Y. 1974.

Klevay, L.M: Hair as a Biopsy Material. **Arch.Intern.Med.** 138, 1978.

Mahler, D.J, Scott, A.F., Walsh, J.R., Haynie, G: A Study of Trace Metals in Fingernails and Hair Using Neutron Activation Analysis. **J.Nuc.Med.** 12, 1970.

Sauberlich, H.E., Dowdy, R.P., Skala, J.H: **Laboratory Tests for the Assessment of Nutritional Status.** CRC Press, Fl. 1984.

EPA 600/3-80-089, 1980.

Clin. Chem., 36,3, 1990.

Chatt, A., Katz, S.A: **Hair Analysis Applications in the Biomedical and Environmental Sciences.** VCH Pub, N.Y. 1988.

Am. J. Clin. Nutr, 1978.

Valkovic, V: **Human Hair Trace Element Levels, Vol.II.** CRC Press, Fl. 1988.

Am. J. Epidem., 1977.

Chapter 2

Nutritional Relationships

Did you know that taking too much iron can contribute to certain types of cancers, but too little iron can also have the same effect? Or, that calcium can help prevent osteoporosis, the brittle bones disease, but calcium supplements can also contribute to brittle bones in some people? Or that iron deficiency can cause anemia, but taking too much iron can also cause a certain type of anemia?

As you can see, the field of nutrition can be complex and confusing. The key to understanding the effect of nutrients is to understand their interrelationships. Their relationships are like an interlocking gear system. When a single mineral in the body is affected, either too much or too little, it can have an effect upon at least two other minerals, which in turn will affect two others, etc. For example, a deficiency of vitamin C can allow the mineral copper to build up in the body to the point of toxicity. Too much copper in turn can cause an iron, selenium, or potassium deficiency. Too much vitamin C on the other hand can cause a copper deficiency and result in too much iron retention.

Synergistic And Antagonistic Relationships

There are two basic relationships that exist between nutrients. In some instances they work together or in cooperation with each other. This is called a synergistic relationship. At other times nutrients can work against each other. This is called an antagonistic relationship.

Nutrients work synergistically or cooperatively within the cell on a metabolic level. They also may aid absorption from the intestinal tract. The minerals iron and copper, for example, are closely related, and are needed by the body in the right proportions for production of red blood cells. Without enough copper, iron could not be incorporated into hemoglobin. Magnesium may be required to correct potassium deficiency symptoms, since magnesium enhances the cellular retention of potassium. Calcium, magnesium, and phosphorus work together to maintain the skeletal structures. Vitamin C helps with the intestinal absorption of iron, and vitamin D enhances calcium absorption.

Antagonism of nutrients also occurs at the intestinal or cellular level. For example, if we consume an excessive amount of calcium in our diet, it can result in decreased absorption of zinc, iron, phosphorus, and magnesium. As mentioned previously, iron and copper are a pair that work together. However, too much iron can inhibit the absorption of copper, and of course too much copper can interfere with iron absorption. Iron and copper can also interfere with each other on a metabolic level. Iron excess within the cell can adversely affect the metabolic functions of copper and vise versa.

Mineral Interrelationships - Antagonism

Figure 2 is a mineral wheel showing the antagonistic relationship between minerals. Calcium (Ca) at the top of the chart has a line drawn to magnesium (Mg) at the bottom of the chart. Arrows point toward calcium and magnesium indicating a mutual antagonism. We can also see a line from calcium to phosphorus (P), with arrows pointing in both directions. This would indicate that too much calcium can contribute to a magnesium or phosphorus deficiency, and too much magnesium or phosphorus can contribute to a calcium deficiency.

Nutritional Relationships

Figure 2
Mineral Antagonisms

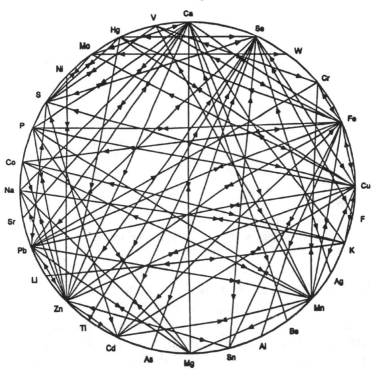

Calcium (Ca)	Selenium (Se)	Chromium (Cr)	Iron (Fe)
Copper (Cu)	Potassium (K)	Manganese (Mn)	Aluminum (Al)
Magnesium (Mg)	Cadmium (Cd)	Zinc (Zn)	Lead (Pb)
Sodium (Na)	Phosphorus (P)	Nickel (Ni)	Mercury (Hg)
Vanadium (V)	Molybdenum (Mo)	Sulfur (S)	Cobalt (Co)
Strontium (Sr)	Lithium (Li)	Thallium (Tl)	Arsenic (As)
Tin (Sn)		Beryllium (Be)	Silver (Ag)
Fluorine (F)			

Mineral Synergism

The following list represents some of the mineral synergisms. A number of the synergistic minerals are also shown to be antagonistic in the mineral wheel. This illustrates the delicate balance among minerals. Even though phosphorus and calcium are antagonistic, they also work together. In the proper balance they maintain the integrity of the bones and teeth.

MINERAL	SYNERGISTIC MINERALS
Calcium	Magnesium-Phosphorus-Copper-Sodium-Potassium-Selenium
Magnesium	Calcium-Potassium-Zinc-Manganese-Phosphorus-Chromium
Sodium	Potassium-Selenium-Cobalt-Calcium-Copper-Phosphorus-Iron
Potassium	Sodium-Magnesium-Cobalt-Manganese-Zinc-Phosphorus-Iron
Copper	Iron-Cobalt-Calcium-Sodium-Selenium
Zinc	Potassium-Magnesium-Manganese-Chromium-Phosphorus
Phosphorus	Calcium-Magnesium-Sodium-Zinc-Potassium-Iron
Iron	Copper-Manganese-Potassium-Sodium-Chromium-Phosphorus-Selenium
Chromium	Magnesium-Zinc-Potassium
Manganese	Potassium-Zinc-Magnesium-Iron-Phosphorus
Selenium	Sodium-Potassium-Copper-Iron-Manganese-Calcium

Vitamin Interrelationships - Antagonism

As with minerals, a similar relationship exists among the vitamins. Figure 3 is a wheel showing some of the antagonism between vitamins. As an example, a line is drawn from vitamin A to vitamin E with arrows pointing both directions. This illustrates that excess amounts of vitamin A can contribute to a vitamin E deficiency, or at the very least, increase its requirements. Too much vitamin E similarly affects vitamin A. Known antagonism between vitamins is indicated by solid lines while theoretical antagonisms are indicated by broken lines.

Figure 3
Vitamin Antagonisms

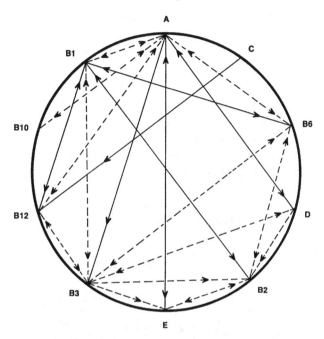

Vitamin Synergism

The following chart shows a partial list of vitamin synergists. The vitamins work together and can even protect against deficiency symptoms, or spare another vitamin that may not be adequate in the diet.

VITAMIN	VITAMIN SYNERGISTS
A	$C-E-B_1-B_2-B_3-B_6$
D	$E-B_{12}$
E	$A-C-B_1-B_3-B_5-B_6-B_{10}-B_{12}$
B_1	$A-E-C-B_2-B_3-B_5-B_6-B_{10}-B_{12}$
B_2	$A-B_3-B_{10}$
B_6	$A-E-B_1-B_3-B_5-B_{10}-B_{12}$
B_{12}	$C-D-E-B_1-B_3-B_5-B_6-B_{10}$
C	$A-E-B_3-B_5-B_6$
B_3	$A-E-B_1-B_2-B_5-B_6-B_{10}$
B_5	$A-C-E-B_1-B_3-B_6-B_{10}$

Vitamin-Mineral Interrelationships - Antagonism

Even though vitamins and minerals work together in the body, excessive intake of a single vitamin can lead to mineral imbalances by producing a deficiency, or by increasing the retention of a mineral. For instance, high vitamin C intake can contribute to a copper deficiency and yet cause excessive iron retention. Vitamin D can increase calcium absorption and retention, but too much can cause a potassium deficiency. Excessive intake of a mineral can also increase or decrease the requirement of a vitamin. Too much copper in the body is known to increase vitamin C and niacin requirements. Other vitamin-mineral antagonisms are shown in the vitamin-mineral wheel in figure 4.

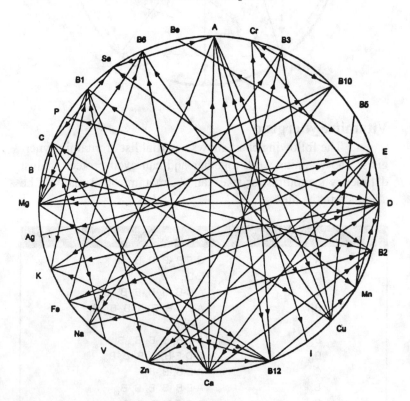

Figure 4
Vitamin-Mineral Antagonisms

Vitamin-Mineral Synergism

Vitamins are closely associated with the metabolic functions of minerals. Enzymes are proteins that initiate cellular metabolic processes and require minerals for their activation. Vitamins are considered co-enzymes, aiding the minerals in their activity. Vitamin supplementation may be required in order to correct a mineral deficiency. A classic example is rickets, a calcium disorder in children, which responds readily to vitamin D supplementation. Both vitamins C and A may be required to correct iron deficiency anemia. Zinc provides another good example. The body requires zinc for vitamin A to be mobilized from storage areas in order for it to be utilized by other tissues. If a zinc deficiency is present, a person can have plenty of vitamin A in the liver and yet have signs of vitamin A deficiency. In studies of individuals suffering from night blindness, a classic sign of vitamin A deficiency, they found that many would not improve after being given vitamin A supplements. Those patients that did not respond were found to have a co-existing zinc deficiency. When zinc was given, the night blindness was corrected. In this situation, taking more vitamin A could produce a nutritional imbalance between other vitamins and minerals.

The following is a partial list of vitamin-mineral synergists:

VITAMIN	MINERAL SYNERGISTS
A	Zinc-Potassium-Phosphorus-Selenium-Magnesium-Manganese
B_1	Selenium-Cobalt-Sodium-Potassium-Iron-Manganese-Phosphorus-Magnesium-Copper-Zinc
B_2	Iron-Phosphorus-Magnesium-Zinc-Potassium-Chromium
B_3	Zinc-Potassium-Iron-Phosphorus-Magnesium-Manganese-Sodium-Chromium-Selenium
B_5	Chromium-Sodium-Potassium-Zinc-Phosphorus
B_6	Zinc-Chromium-Magnesium-Sodium-Potassium-Phosphorus-Iron-Manganese-Selenium
B_{12}	Selenium-Copper-Calcium-Cobalt-Sodium
C	Iron-Copper-Manganese-Zinc-Selenium-Phosphorus-Magnesium
D	Calcium-Magnesium-Sodium-Copper-Selenium
E	Sodium-Potassium-Calcium-Iron-Manganese-Zinc-Phosphorus-Selenium

Conclusion

These nutritional relationships help to explain why people may respond so differently to nutritional therapy and supplementation. With the use of dietary supplements it is not uncommon to see nutritionally induced deficiencies. This is often caused by the large intake of single vitamins or minerals.

As an example, many people take large dosages of vitamin C to help prevent or alleviate the symptoms of a cold or the flu. This does help, but one should be aware of the copper lowering effect of vitamin C. If you lose too much copper, you may be helping to prevent viruses, but you could be making yourself more susceptible to bacterial infections.

Excessive vitamin E intake can produce symptoms that suggest a vitamin A deficiency. Taking vitamin A will counteract the effects of vitamin E, but could eventually produce a vitamin D deficiency.

One of the most abused nutrients is the mineral calcium. Even the young are taking calcium supplements to prevent the development of brittle bones when they get older. Little concern is given to the potential side effects of these megadoses. Individuals taking too much calcium may be causing a deficiency of phosphorus and magnesium, thereby contributing to the very condition they are trying to prevent.

When it comes to vitamin and mineral interactions, nutrition involves more than eating three meals a day, relying on the four food groups, or randomly taking supplements. They are all essential to good health, but taking the time to learn how they function together may be just as essential to our health.

References

Davies, I: **The Clinical Significance of the Essential Biological Metals.** M.B. London, 1921.
Prasad, A.S.: **Trace Elements and Iron in Human Metabolism.** Plenum Pub., N.Y., 1978.
Allen R: Abstracts. **18th Congress of The International Society of Hematology.** Monterey Ca., Aug, 1980.
Clark and Basset: **J. Exp. Med.,** 115, 147, 1982.
Pollack S., George, J.N., Reba, R.C., Kaufman, R.M., Crosby, W.H: The Absorption of Non-ferrous Metals in Iron Deficiency. **J.Clin.Invest.,** 44, 1965.
Forth, W., Rummel, W: Absorption of Iron and Chemically Related Metals in vitro and in vivo: Specificity of Iron Binding System in the Mucosa of the Jejunum. **Intestinal Absorption of Metal Ions, Trace Elements and Radionuclides.** Skoryna, S.C., Waldron-Edward, D., Eds. Pergamon Press, N.Y., 1971.
Valberg, L.S., Ludwig, J., Olatubosun, D: Alteration in Cobalt Absorption in Patients with Disorders of Iron Metabolism. **Gastroent.,** 56, 1969.
White, Handler, Smith: **Principles of Biochemistry,** 3rd Ed. McGraw Hill, N.Y., 1964.
Kleiner and Orten: **Biochemistry,** 6th Ed. Mosby, St.Louis, Mo. 1962.
Kutsky, R.J: **Handbook of Vitamins, Minerals, and Hormones,** 2nd Ed. Van Norstrand Reinhold Co., N.Y., 1981.
Nutrition Reviews, Present Knowledge in Nutrition, 5th Ed. The Nutr. Found., Inc., Wash., D.C., 1984.
Ciba-Geigy Limited. Basle, Switz., 1970.
Magnesium in Human Nutrition. Home Econ.Res.Rep. No. 19, U.S.D.A. Aug, 1962.
Finley, M.S., Cerklewski, E.L: Influence of Ascorbic Acid Supplementation on Copper Status in Young Adult Men. **Am.J.Clin.Nutr.** 37, 1983.
Smith, J.C: Interrelationship of Zinc and Vitamin A Metabolism in Animal and Human Nutrition: A Review. **Clinical, Biochemical and Nutritional Aspects of Trace Elements.** Prasad, A.S., (ed.) Alan R. Liss, N.Y., 1982.
Mason, K.E: A Conspectus of Research on Copper Metabolism and Requirements of Man. **J.of Nutr.,** 109, 11, 1979.

Chapter 3

Nutritional-Endocrine Relationships

Frequently the terms "diet" and "nutrition" are used interchangeably. However, a vast distinction can be made between the two. Diet describes the consumption of foods, while nutrition describes the nutrients obtained from the diet. It is important to recognize the difference in these terms, since the presence of nutrients in the diet does not necessarily insure their absorption, retention, or utilization by the body. Nutrition is therefore affected or controlled by factors other than diet alone.

Two of these controlling factors include the central nervous system and the endocrine system. Together they are called the neuro-endocrine system. This system is not often taken into consideration when evaluating an individual's nutritional status. However, the neuro-endocrine system has a powerful and far-reaching impact upon the body, affecting absorption, excretion, transport, utilization and storage of nutrients. These include minerals, as well as vitamins, proteins, fats, and carbohydrates.

Sympathetic And Parasympathetic Nervous System

A two way communication exists between the tissues and the central nervous system (CNS). CNS activity affects eating behavior and metabolism by way of sympathetic and parasympathetic nerves. Generally speaking, the sympathetic branch of the nervous system speeds up the activity of the body, while the para-sympathetic branch slows it down. They have an effect upon the rate of organ function, enzyme activity, immunity, and hormone release. For example, sympathetic stimulation to the pancreas causes a decrease in insulin release, but para-sympathetic stimulation increases insulin release. The para-sympathetic and sympathetic branches oppose each other and generally work in concert with the endocrine glands of the body.

The Endocrine Glands

The endocrine system is very complex. First we should look at some of the major endocrine relationships. As with vitamins and minerals, the endocrine glands have an antagonistic and synergistic relationship. Figure 5 shows the hormonal antagonism between some of the endocrine glands and hormones.

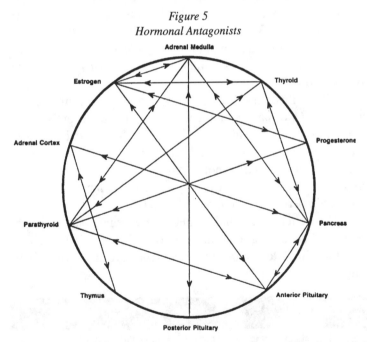

Figure 5
Hormonal Antagonists

As an example, a line is drawn between estrogen and the thyroid. The arrows pointing both directions indicate that over activity of the thyroid gland can suppress estrogen production, and too much estrogen can contribute to low thyroid activity. This may help to explain why some women who begin taking estrogen, or estrogen dominant oral contraceptive agents may develop fatigue, blood sugar disturbance, gain weight, and even experience depression with their low energy levels. Too much estrogen could be a factor in causing these reactions by contributing to hypothyroidism and a corresponding reduction in metabolic rate. This could also explain why the feelings of lethargy, weight gain, and depression occur in women premenstrually. This is the time when estrogen levels begin to rise. If thyroid function is already low, even this normal hormonal fluctuation can cause a problem by further suppressing the thyroid. Perhaps the premenstrual syndrome, or PMS, could more descriptively be termed premenstrual hypothyroidism. Frequently, women who experience problems on estrogen-dominant birth control pills feel much better when their doctor switches them to a progesterone-dominant pill. Progesterone reduces the adverse effects upon the thyroid gland and is considered synergistic to its function. We can also see from the chart that an over active thyroid, or the taking of thyroid stimulants, could adversely affect estrogen status. This could lead to calcium loss and eventually osteoporosis.

This illustrates that rarely does an endocrine problem develop alone. One gland does not become over or under active without affecting another. This would be true with a clinical endocrine disturbance, as well as a sub-clinical endocrine disturbance. In other words, a person does not have to have a pathological condition such as Addison's or Cushings disease to have a disturbed relationship between the endocrine glands.

To better understand the neuro-endocrine system it can be categorized according to stimulating or sedating effects. Table 1 shows the stimulatory sympathetic, and sedative para-sympathetic groups.

Table 1

SYMPATHETIC ENDOCRINE GLANDS	PARA-SYMPATHETIC ENDOCRINE GLANDS
Hypothalmus (Medial protion)	Hypothalamus (Lateral portion)
Anterior Pituitary	Posterior Pituitary
Adrenal Cortex (Catabolic)	Adrenal Cortex (Anabolic)
Adrenal Medulla	Pancreas (Endocrine)
Thyroid	Parathyroid
Ovaries (Progesterone)	Ovaries (Estrogen)

Normally there is somewhat of a balance between these two groups, but actually in healthy individuals the glands constantly vacillate depending upon the circumstance. Hormones from the endocrine glands have many functions within the body, but generally speaking, they regulate metabolic activity by speeding it up or slowing it down. The stimulatory group opposes, or is antagonistic to, the sedative group. For example, when there is a sympathetic neuro-endocrine discharge, the heart rate increases, and the blood pressure goes up. This occurs with an acute stress, such as nearly being involved in an auto accident. The para-sympathetic group eventually intervenes, bringing the heart rate, and blood pressure back to normal. Of course, many other functions in the body are affected as well. These two groups normally keep each other in check. However, if there is a disturbance in their balance one group can become dominant, causing a person's metabolism to become either over-stimulated or too sedated.

Nutritional Effects Of The Neuro-Endocrine System

When the sympathetic neuro-endocrine group is dominant, or over-active, the body will lose essential minerals such as calcium and magnesium. However, other minerals can build up in the body such as sodium, potassium, and phosphorus. This is due to a change in intestinal absorption and reabsorption by the kidneys of these elements. Deficiency of vitamins may also develop due to increased utilization caused by the elevated metabolic rate.

The sympathetic endocrine group can be referred to as the stress glands. They are activated by stress and in turn raise the metabolic rate. This reaction is termed the "fight or flight" mechanism. The nutritional impact of these glands illustrate how some health conditions can flare up when a person is under stress. Some types of high blood pressure, for example, can be stress related due to the increased retention of sodium with a corresponding loss of calcium and magnesium. It is no surprise that researchers have found that calcium and magnesium help lower blood pressure in many people.

The absorption and retention of calcium and magnesium is increased while sodium, potassium, and phosphorus are decreased when the para-sympathetic endocrine group is dominant. When the sedative glands become dominant, a person may begin to feel fatigued, develop low blood pressure, and even suffer from depression. This is largely due to lowered energy production, which is contributed to by the increase in retention of sedative minerals such as calcium and magnesium.

Factors Affecting Endocrine Activity

Normal physiological responses affect the endocrine system and thus nutritional requirements. For example, during pregnancy, an expectant mother will go through major endocrine changes that in turn affect her nutritional requirements. Nursing mothers also have increased nutritional requirements. Infants and children have different nutritional needs during their growth and development compared to an adult.

Stress affects the neuro-endocrine system and nutritional requirements. Stress can be caused by many factors including viral or bacterial infections, or any active disease process, as well as emotions. Toxic metals and chemical exposures also are stressors to the body. Side effects from medications can be considered a stress, since many drugs are known to cause increased excretion, or retention of nutrients. Even athletic performance is considered a stress. Olympic or professional athletes are constantly stressing themselves during training and competition. Their nutritional requirements are usually higher than the average individual.

During the early stage of stress the body normally responds with an alarm reaction. This alarm reaction consists of a sympathetic nervous system discharge that acts as a signal, alerting the neuro-endocrine and immune system of an assault. This results in a heightened metabolic rate. As mentioned previously, this stage of stress is also called the "fight or flight" mechanism. Not only are the minerals affected by this stress reaction, but the utilization of certain vitamins is also increased. Prolonged stress can therefore result in severe nutritional deficiencies including minerals and vitamins.

The alarm stage of stress is usually followed by the resistance stage and then the recovery stage. During each of these stages different hormones secreted from the endocrine glands become involved. At the same time, specific nutrients are also required. Below is a partial list of the nutrients involved in the three stages of stress.

Nutrients Involved In The Alarm Stage Of Stress

VITAMINS	MINERALS
C	Calcium
D	Copper
E	Cobalt
B_1	Sodium
B_6	Selenium
B_{12}	

Nutrients Involved In The Resistance Stage Of Stress

VITAMINS	MINERALS
C	Potassium
A	Zinc
B_1	Manganese
B_2	Iron
B_3	Magnesium
B_5	
B_6	

Nutrients Required In The Recovery Stage Of Stress

VITAMINS	MINERALS
C	Calcium
D	Magnesium
E	Copper
B_1	Cobalt
B_6	Selenium
B_{12}	
Folic Acid	

These stages of stress are a normal reaction by the body. Typically there is a progression from the alarm stage to the recovery stage. However, in some cases, a person may be unable to progress from one stage to the other. If this occurs, then the particular stage that develops can produce disease. As an example, if the alarm stage develops and does not proceed to the resistance stage, then chronic inflammation can set in. This may result in arthritis, colitis, gastritis, etc. The resistant stage can cause extensive destruction throughout the body and result in chronic degenerative disease and even cancer. As mentioned previously, the recovery phase is hopefully reached and is the last stage of the stress reaction. However, if a severe nutritional imbalance occurs, then a person may not recover, but instead may go into an exhaustion stage. This is often referred to as a "burn-out." In other words, the stimulatory glands become weakened to the point that the sedative glands become totally dominant.

The following table summarizes some of the mineral relationships or ratios affected by various endocrine glands.

Table 2

ENDOCRINE	MINERAL RATIOS INCREASED	MINERAL RATIOS DECREASED
Parathyroid	Ca/P - Ca/Mg - Ca/Na Ca/K - Ca/Fe	Fe/Cu
Thyroid	Na/Mg - Fe/Cu	Ca/P - Ca/K
Adrenal Cortex (Anabolic)	Na/K - Na/Mg - Fe/Cu Ca/Mg	Ca/P - Ca/K - Ca/Na
Adrenal Cortex (Catabolic)	Fe/Cu - Na/Mg	Na/K - Ca/K - Ca/P Ca/Mg - Ca/Na
Pancreas	Ca/P - Ca/Mg - Ca/K Ca/Fe - Ca/Na	Zn/Cu - Fe/Cu
Estrogen	Ca/Mg - Ca/P - Ca/K Ca/Na - Ca/Fe - Na/K	Zn/Cu - Fe/Cu
Progesterone	Zn/Cu - Fe/Cu	Na/K - Ca/K

It should also be noted that not only can the endocrine glands affect nutrition, but nutrition can have an effect upon the endocrine glands as well. For example, if a magnesium deficiency develops, certain hormones produced by the adrenal cortex will be increased. Of course, if over-production of this hormone occurs initially, then it will produce a magnesium deficiency. However, when adequate magnesium is restored in the diet this excess hormone production will decrease.

How this information applies to an individual will be discussed in the following chapter.

References

White, Handler, Smith: **Principles of Biochemistry,** 3rd Ed. McGraw Hill, N.Y., 1964.
Kleiner and Orten: **Biochemistry,** 6th Ed. Mosby, St.Louis, Mo. 1962.
Kutsky, R.J: **Handbook of Vitamins, Minerals, and Hormones,** 2nd Ed. Van Norstrand Reinhold Co., N.Y., 1981.
Magnesium in Human Nutrition. Home Econ.Res.Rep. No. 19, U.S.D.A. Aug, 1962.
Henkin, R.I: Trace Metals in Endocrinology. **The Medical Clinics of North America,** 60, 4, 1976.
Pottenger, F.M: **Symptoms of Visceral Disease,** 4th Ed. Mosby Co., St. Louis, Mo. 1930.
Page, M.E: **Degeneration Regeneration.** Nutr. Dev. St.Petersburg Beach, Fl. 1949.
Page, M.E: **Body Chemistry in Health and Disease.** Nutr.Dev. St.Petersburg Beach, Fl.
Rosa, R.M., Silva, P., Young, J.B: Adrenegeric Modulation of Extrarenal Potassium Disposal. **New. Eng. J. Med.,** 302, 1980.
Silva, P., Spokes, K: Sympathetic System in Potassium Homeostasis. **Am. J. Physiol.** 241, 1981.
Guyton, A.C: **Textbook of Medical Physiology,** 4th Ed. Saunders Pub., 1971.
Clark, I., Geoffroy, R.F., Bowers, W: Effects of Adrenal Cortical Steroids on Calcium Metabolism. **Endocrinol.,** 64, 1959.
Kleeman, C.R., Levi, J., Better, O: Kidney and Adrenal-Cortical Hormones. **Nephron.,** 25, 1975.
Mader, I.J., Iseri, L.T: Spontaneous Hypopotassemia, Hypo-Magnesemia, Alkalosis and Tetany Due to Hypersecretion of Corticosterone-Like Mineralcorticoids. **Am. J. Med.,** 19, 1955.
Klim, R.G., et al: Intestinal Calcium Absorption in Exogenous Hypercorticism. Role of 25 (OH) and Corticosteroid Dose.**J. Clin. Invest.,** 60, 1977.
Douglas, W.W., Rubin, R.P: Effects of Alkaline Earths and Other Divalent Cations on Adrenal Medullary Secretion. **J. Physiol.** 175, 1964.
Adams, D., et al: Parathyroid Function in Spontaneous Primary Hypothyroidism. **J. Endocrinol.** 40, 1968.

Chapter 4

Metabolic Individuality

To further understand the field of nutrition it is important to understand some basic concepts. The foremost is the recognition of individuality. While fingerprints set individuals apart from each other, people have another characteristic that makes them unique as well: their metabolism. The late Dr. Roger Williams was one of the earliest researchers to recognize this characteristic, which he called "biochemical individuality."

Genetic studies have shown that a vast diversity exists among the human population. There is also a high degree of variability in the biochemical makeup of individuals that affects their nutritional status, including absorption, excretion, and metabolism of nutrients. Dr. Williams pointed out that adults of the same age and size in similar environmental settings who ate a similar diet, had several-fold differences in their nutritional requirements. Even children within the same family have different biochemical make ups, creating distinct differences in their nutritional needs.

Today there is a greater recognition and acceptance of the fact that metabolic individuality exists. People are being classified according to personality and body types. High stress individuals for example are classified as type A personalities, and are known to be susceptible to stress related diseases. Type B personalities on the other hand, are not as likely to succumb to conditions that affect type A's. Body types are also used to categorize individuals. For example, individuals who have an apple-shaped body structure are found to be susceptible to diabetes, heart disease, and certain types of cancer. The apple shape is due to increased fat deposition in the abdominal region. Individuals with a pear-shaped body structure on the other hand, are not at as much risk for these conditions. Pear-shaped individuals tend to accumulate fat below the hips, in the buttocks and thighs.

To determine if you have an apple or pear shaped body type, measure your hips and waist. Then divide your waist measurement by your hip measurement. If the result is 0.75 or less you have a pear shaped body type. If the result is greater than 0.75 you have a tendency toward an apple shape.

Other means of classifying individuals include blood types and even height. Emerging data is beginning to reveal that people are susceptible to health conditions depending on how tall or short they are. Reports have even suggested that right handed people have a longer life span than left handed people.

Tissue Mineral Analysis And Metabolic Types

"If any facet of an individual's life history leaves a biochemical mark that can be measured in the laboratory, then this life history marker can potentially be used to specify individuality." Based upon this statement, a plausible model for determining metabolic types can be presented through mineral patterns found in biopsied human hair. The study of thousands of TMAs has revealed distinctive patterns which help to recognize metabolic types.

Eight metabolic categories can be identified through properly obtained, assayed and interpreted hair samples. These include the fast metabolic types 1 through 4, and the slow metabolic types 1 through 4. People generally fall into these two categories: they are either "fast" or "slow" metabolizers.

The term metabolism describes the utilization of nutrients and the efficiency of that utilization on a cellular level. The neurological and endocrine systems largely govern cellular metabolism and nutritional status. One's nutritional status in turn also affects these systems.

There are telltale signs that distinguish fast from slow metabolizers. They appear depending upon the degree of trace element imbalances, endocrine activity, and how long the pattern has been present.

The Fast Metabolizer

The fast metabolizer's thyroid and adrenal glands work overtime, accelerating cellular metabolic activity. One by-product of this increased work load is heat. A fast metabolizer usually feels warm and may perspire very easily. They can start sweating even while they are doing very little physical labor. Just eating a meal can cause them to break out in perspiration.

Fast metabolizers are typically cerebral sorts who are intellectually oriented. Often their mental activity is undirected; they often jump from subject to subject. They are often hyper and have a difficult time relaxing. If their metabolism becomes excessive, they may become easily agitated. These people often gravitate toward stressful situations and are often referred to as stress-aholics. You probably know one: they start several projects at once, even though it is near impossible to finish them all on time. They wait until the last minute to meet deadlines. More often than not, they are late for appointments, even though they have every intention of being on time. This type of individual has been labeled as having a "type A" personality.

Fast metabolizers also have big egos. They enjoy being the center of attention and feel this is appropriate, since they view themselves and their work of utmost importance. Being late for appointments is probably an unconscious way of drawing attention to himself/herself and increases their sense of importance.

Because they view themselves as competent and capable, fast metabolizers believe their work is critically important. There is no one who can do their job; they are irreplaceable, in their view. Therefore, they have a difficult time delegating duties to others. Fast metabolizers can be difficult to work for, and even live with, and demand perfection from those around them. They, however, do not have the biochemical makeup conducive to having the patience required to be perfect.

They can rarely find time for a vacation because their work is the driving force of their lives. Taking time off to sit on a beach in Aruba would seem boring and senseless. These folks generally refuse to waste time at social gatherings unless they can dominate the group by being the center of attention. Since they consider themselves the most important person at the party, they often talk incessantly without letting others get a word in edgewise. However, they use their loquaciousness to cover up their feelings of shyness and inadequacy. Being on the fast track of constant stress also helps them avoid introspection or having to admit their inadequacy. They have great difficulties planning for the future. If they look too far ahead, they become very anxious.

The fast metabolizers frequently develop addictive personality traits, and often become obsessive and compulsive. They can easily become addicted to substance abuse such as alcohol, and even foods.

Many of their character traits can be traced to hyperglycemia, or high blood sugar. When the blood sugar is higher than normal they can become euphoric. When their blood sugar drops below normal, they become even more stressed and irritable. The irritability or anger is even a fix, because it stimulates the adrenals which in turn helps to raise their blood sugar. Their metabolic mineral pattern can cause them to become sensitive to noises, develop fine muscle tremors, or cramps, and have difficulty falling asleep easily. They often describe themselves as night owls. Their metabolism increases their susceptibility to cardiovascular disease, peptic ulcers, histamine allergies, arthritis, and diabetes. This metabolic pattern also causes them to put on weight in the torso, or abdominal region. This gives them the characteristic apple-shaped body structure.

Factors Contributing To Fast Metabolism

Several factors cause a person to become a fast metabolizer. Quite often children inherit their mineral patterns from their parents. However, almost all children are born with a fast metabolic rate. This is nature's way of ensuring they have the resources for a constant and quick growth rate. However, a family's eating habits will cement that fast rate, or slow it considerably, making it a permanent feature of their offspring's biochemistry. We find most teenagers share their parents' trace element patterns.

Genetic similarity, combined with similar environmental influences, help explain how certain health conditions are passed from one generation to the next. Children with the same mineral patterns as their parents will be predisposed to similar health conditions and even personality traits.

Stress is another major influence. A stressful lifestyle increases the metabolic rate. Stress causes the body to retain the minerals that stimulate and excite, while losing the nutrients conducive to quiet and calm. If a fast metabolizer experiences a period of prolonged stress, the results can be disastrous. A vicious cycle develops as the body slowly loses its ability to calm itself due to an inability to adequately store sedative minerals.

Slow Metabolism

Approximately 80 percent of the American population are slow metabolizers. They are a mirror image of their hurry-up counterparts. Unlike fast metabolizers, their calcium and magnesium levels are much higher in relation to phosphorus, sodium and potassium. Their parathyroid and pancreatic hormones work overtime, and their thyroid and adrenal glands become sluggish. This results in a slowing down of the cellular metabolic activity, and accumulation of sedative minerals.

The slow metabolizer has a tendency to gain weight in the hips and thighs, creating a pear-shaped silhouette. Slow metabolizers generally have low blood pressure. They frequently develop postural hypotension, a condition that causes the blood pressure to drop when getting up from a lying, or sitting position. If the adrenal glands cannot react fast enough to the change in position, the slow metabolizer will feel dizzy. Their heart rate also tends to be slow, but can be punctuated with intermittent periods of rapid heartbeats.

Slow metabolizers may tire easily, thanks to their slow glandular activity. The reduced glandular activity can also retard circulation, resulting in a reduced blood flow to the extremities. Slow metabolizers also suffer from low body temperature. This increases their sensitivity to cold, which they notice particularly in their hands and feet.

These metabolizers may also develop Type II insomnia, which is a malady that can destroy top performance. They can fall asleep easily, but awaken frequently throughout the night. They wake up feeling tired, even after they've been asleep 10 to 12 hours. This restless sleep contributes to their constant fatigue. Ironically, they develop this trouble because they don't have enough energy. Restful sleep requires energy to reach the stage of rejuvenating rest, which is characterized by rapid eye movement (REM). When the state of REM sleep is not maintained long enough, fatigue will eventually become chronic.

Increased insulin levels can contribute to hypoglycemia, which is also associated with fatigue. Depression frequently accompanies the fatigue. People with slow metabolism perform like the perfectionists the fast metabolizers would like to be. They have the ability to follow a complicated project through to completion. Emotionally, they may face major hurdles expressing their deeper emotions. They may suffer from low self-esteem and feelings of inferiority.

It is inescapable that our emotions are closely related to our body chemistry. How we feel about ourselves, our colleagues and loved ones, as well as the world around us can be translated into chemical equations. As alcoholics and drug addicts know so well, we can alter these emotions and replace them with others by simply changing our body chemistry. Energy levels have a profound effect on our emotions. The higher our energy level, the more positive, optimistic and self-assured we become. If our energy stores are low, we can become depressed and pessimistic.

Factors Contributing To A Slow Metabolic Rate

Genetic makeup plays a major role in the metabolic rate, but eating habits also occupy center stage in controlling that rate. Most vegetarians for example, have a slow metabolic rate. A viral infection will also reduce cellular activity. If the infection is vicious enough, for instance, it can have the strength to convert a fast metabolizer to a slow metabolizer, as a by-product of suppressing the invading organism. Yeast and fungus infections also reduce the metabolic rate. Tests of individuals who suffer Chronic Fatigue Syndrome, or who have a virus such as Epstein Barr, and/

or cytomegleo virus, as well as candida (yeast infection), invariably show slow TMA profiles.

Manifestations of the emotional and physical characteristics of the fast and slow metabolizer type 1's depend upon a number of factors. These include the degree or severity of the trace element imbalances (including vitamins and amino acids), endocrine activity, and the length of time the imbalance has been present.

The subtypes 2 through 4 have variations of these characteristics. Each type of metabolism has advantages and disadvantages. One type is not necessarily better than the other. Here the golden mean is the best. It is best to strike a nutrient balance, whether in a slow or fast metabolic category.

It is possible to change the body chemistry and step up the metabolic process from slow to fast, and vice-versa. But, personality changes usually accompany a change in metabolism. A person must be willing to go through the personality reversals that are by-products of the new body chemistry.

The graph of the slow metabolizer in figure 6 shows the increased retention of sedative minerals relative to stimulatory minerals. This is a result of a relative overactivity of the sedative neuro-endocrine system. The parathyroid gland is dominant, resulting in increased retention of calcium and magnesium. In turn, if you refer to the endocrine wheel in the previous chapter, you will find that the parathyroid hormone decreases the activity of the thyroid. Decreased thyroid activity contributes to this mineral pattern and reduced metabolic rate. Typically when the thyroid gland is low, the adrenal activity is also reduced. This is reflected in the low tissue levels of sodium and potassium. Further, copper, a sedative mineral, is an antagonist to the thyroid and contributes to a reduced metabolic rate.

The fast metabolic graph, shown in figure 7, indicates the dominance of stimulatory minerals relative to low levels of sedative minerals. Dominance of the sympathetic neuro-endocrine group results in an increase in sodium, potassium, phosphorus, and iron, and decreased levels of calcium, magnesium, copper and zinc. This pattern indicates an increase in adrenal and thyroid activity by high tissue levels of sodium and potassium. These stimulatory glands in turn antagonize the sedative glands, such as the parathyroid and pancreas.

Figure 6
Slow Metabolic Mineral Pattern

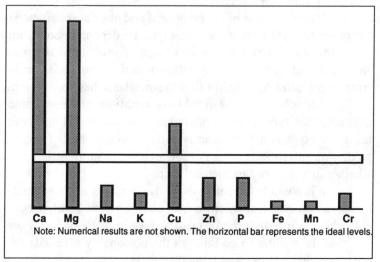

Figure 7
Fast Metabolic Mineral Pattern

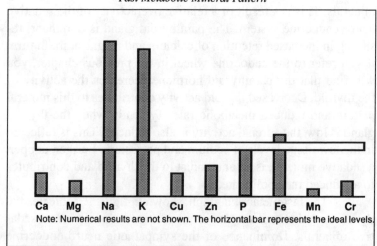

Advantage Of Knowing One's Metabolic Type

There are several advantages to knowing one's metabolic type. As discussed previously, we know that individuals are subject to specific health conditions depending upon their personality such as type A or B, and body types such as apple or pear shapes. Body types, personality types and metabolic types are all affected by the body chemistry. Body chemistry is of course affected or controlled by the endocrine and nervous systems. These systems also affect nutritional status. Conversely, these systems can be changed through specific nutritional factors.

Classification Of Disease Processes

Optimum or ideal health would consist of a well-balanced neuro-endocrine system. This in turn would provide a well-balanced body chemistry. An improper or unbalanced neuro-endocrine system will lead to nutritional imbalances that will eventually lead to less than optimum health.

Many health conditions can be classified according to overstimulation of a branch of the neuro-endocrine system. An increased or excessively stimulated metabolic rate is due to increased sympathetic activity. When the para-sympathetic system becomes too active, the metabolic rate becomes sluggish or overly sedated. The result is a specific change in one's body chemistry, which inevitably affects one's nutritional status and requirements.

The following is a partial list of conditions that have been categorized according to too much sympathetic and para-sympathetic activity. This list has been compiled as a result of clinical research and evaluation of more than 250,000 TMA profiles submitted by doctors from throughout the United States. This is not a complete list by any means, and of course, there are always exceptions. The reason for the exceptions is that there is more than one cause for a particular condition. For example, hypertension is largely attributed to a sympathetic condition. Too much stimulation from the sympathetic system does contribute to high blood pressure. However, since there are several factors that can cause high blood pressure, the condition may also be found in individuals who are para-sympathetic dominant, due to completely different reasons.

Conditions Associated With Sympathetic Dominance

Anxiety	Arthritis (rheumatoid)
Allergies (histamine)	A.L.S.
Hypertension	Hyperthyroidism
Hyperadrenia	Hodgkin's disease
Leukemia	Infections (bacterial)
Multiple Sclerosis	Parkinson's Disease
Ulcers (peptic or duodenal)	Diabetes (juvenile)
Increased Humoral Immune Response	

Conditions Associated With Para-sympathetic Dominance

Arthritis (osteo type)	Allergies (low histamine)
Asthma	A.I.D.S.
Anorexia	Fungus
Hypotension	Hypothyroidism
Hypoadrenia	Infections (viral)
Lupus	P.M.S.
Yeast infections	Ulcers (gastric)
Diabetes (adult onset)	Increased Cellular Immune Response

Classification Of Nutrients - Vitamins And Minerals

Minerals can be classified according to their stimulating or sedating effects upon the neuro-endocrine system. Vitamins can also be categorized due to their influence upon mineral metabolism and absorption. A person who has a fast metabolic rate, for example, should avoid excessive intake of the stimulatory nutrients. Instead, they should focus on supplementing with the sedative nutrients. This is why many individuals report feeling nervous and jittery when taking a supplement containing high amounts of the stimulatory B-complex vitamins. Other examples involve vitamin E. In some cases, vitamin E will raise blood pressure. This is why caution is suggested when supplementing with large amounts of vitamin E in individuals who have high blood pressure. Calcium, vitamin D and vitamin B_{12} are considered sedative to the thyroid gland. Their use should be evaluated according to one's thyroid efficiency. These nutrients would be considered very beneficial for the fast metabolic type, but could further sedate a slow metabolism.

The following is a partial list of nutrients that stimulate or sedate the body's metabolic processes.

STIMULATING NUTRIENTS	SEDATIVE NUTRIENTS
Vitamin A	Vitamin B_2
Vitamin B_1	Vitamin B_{12}
Vitamin B_3	Vitamin D
Vitamin B_5	Calcium
Vitamin B_6	Magnesium
Vitamin B_{10}	Zinc
Vitamin E	Copper
Phosphorus	Chromium
Sodium	
Potassium	
Iron	
Manganese	
Selenium	

Water

Even water can be classified as being stimulatory or sedative and can therefore have a positive or negative effect upon our total health. Hard water, for example, is classified as being sedative, and has a high amount of calcium and magnesium relative to sodium and potassium. As you recall, calcium and magnesium are sedative minerals. Hard water is also alkaline.

Soft water on the other hand, is stimulatory. Soft water is acidic compared to hard water, and the mineral pattern is opposite to the mineral pattern of hard water. Calcium and magnesium levels are very low relative to sodium and potassium. Several studies have confirmed that death rates from cardiovascular disease are higher in areas with soft water. The fast metabolic type, especially if he or she is experiencing health problems associated with sympathetic dominance, such as high blood pressure, should avoid soft water in favor of hard water.

Figure 8
Mineral Analysis Pattern of Hard Water

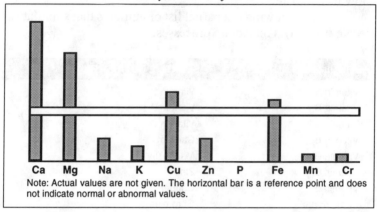

Note: Actual values are not given. The horizontal bar is a reference point and does not indicate normal or abnormal values.

Figure 9
Mineral Analysis Pattern of Soft Water.

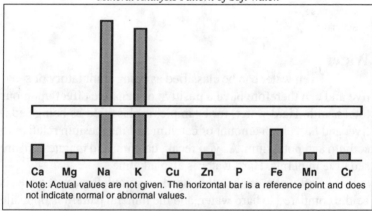

Note: Actual values are not given. The horizontal bar is a reference point and does not indicate normal or abnormal values.

Slow metabolic types may consider using soft water for drinking purposes. The stimulatory effect of soft water would help in raising one's metabolic rate, but should not present a cardiovascular risk.

Foods

Foods can influence the metabolic rate in several ways. They can be classified into stimulatory or sedative categories due to: their 1) Specific Dynamic Action (SDA); 2) Naturally occurring substances that inhibit mineral absorption; and 3) Mineral and vitamin dominance of individual foods.

SDA is a term used to describe the metabolic stimulating effects of foods. All foods increase the metabolic rate to some extent, but some more than others. Foods having the lowest to highest SDA include fats, carbohydrates, and protein.

Eating a meal composed largely of fats, for example, produces a stimulation of the metabolic rate only about 4 to 15 percent. Eating a large meal of carbohydrates, such as spaghetti, or pasta increases the metabolic rate a little more than fats, approximately 4 to 30 percent. A large protein meal increases the metabolic rate by 30 to 70 percent. Protein foods have the highest SDA therefore, slow metabolic types would benefit from consuming them. Fast metabolic types, on the other hand, should not consume a great deal of protein, since their metabolic rate is already accelerated. Fat is generally considered as being sedative. Foods high in fat tend to make one sluggish, especially if they have a slow metabolic rate. Chocolate, for example, which is craved by women who have PMS symptoms, often has a calming effect. Chocolate is very high in fat. Dairy foods such as milk and cheese have a reputation of being sedative. A glass of warm milk to help one sleep for instance has been used for hundreds of years. Dairy foods are sedative due to their high calcium content as well as their high fat content. Foods high in fat would prove beneficial for fast metabolic types, but due to their sedative effects, should be avoided by slow metabolic types.

Naturally occurring substances in foods can inhibit the absorption of minerals. For example, oxalic acid is a substance which binds with calcium in the intestinal tract and actually prevents calcium absorption. These foods are spinach, beet greens, rhubarb, and chard. Phytic acid found in cereals and grains have the same effect. Therefore, these foods would be considered stimulating and are recommended for the slow metabolic types, but should be avoided by fast metabolic types.

Some foods are called goitrogens since they contain naturally occurring thyroid inhibiting substances such as cyanogenic glucosides, or thiocyanates. These include brassica and cruciferous plants such as cassava, sorghum, apricots, prunes, cherries, bamboo shoots, cauliflower, broccoli, brussel sprouts, soy and cabbage. These foods should be avoided by the slow metabolic individual but should be increased in the diet of fast metabolic types.

The mineral constituents of foods also affect the metabolic rate. Sodium for example is known in some cases, to contribute to high blood pressure. High sodium foods can therefore be classified as stimulatory. Coffee is considered to be a stimulant due to its caffeine content. However, coffee is very high in stimulatory nutrients such as iron, potassium, manganese, niacin, and thiamin.

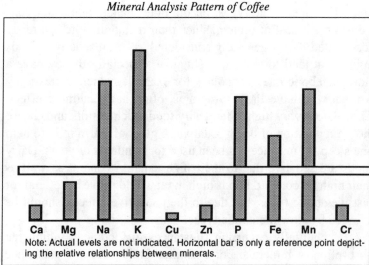

Figure 10
Mineral Analysis Pattern of Coffee

Note: Actual levels are not indicated. Horizontal bar is only a reference point depicting the relative relationships between minerals.

The mineral pattern of salted pretzels is shown on the following page indicating a stimulatory pattern of mineral levels.

Figure 11
Mineral pattern of Pretzel (salted)

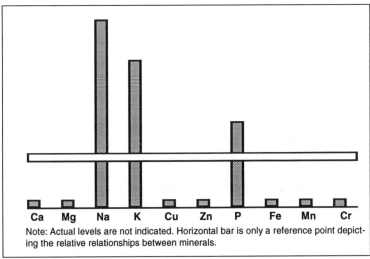

Cola drinks contain sugar and caffeine, but apart from this, it is obvious from the mineral pattern that it can be considered stimulatory. We can see why some children with a fast metabolic rate could become more hyperactive after drinking colas.

Figure 12
Mineral pattern of popular Cola Drink (regular sweetened)

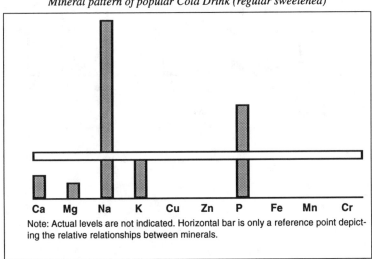

Herbs

There are many constituents found in herbs that give them their unique properties. However, herbs may also be classified as being stimulatory or sedative based upon their mineral content. The following figures show the mineral pattern of some common herbs we have analyzed. It should be noted that the mineral content of herbs can vary considerably, due to the mineral content of the soils in which they have been grown, as well as how they have been processed.

The herb licorice is frequently recommended to increase energy and is known to have adrenal supporting effects. The principle active ingredient is attributed to glycyrrhizic acid, but the mineral pattern found in licorice root is very high in the stimulatory minerals sodium, potassium, iron, and manganese.

Figure 13
Mineral Pattern Of Licorice Root

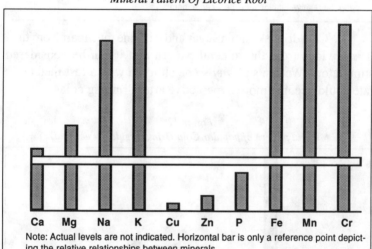

Figure 14
Mineral Pattern Of Ginseng

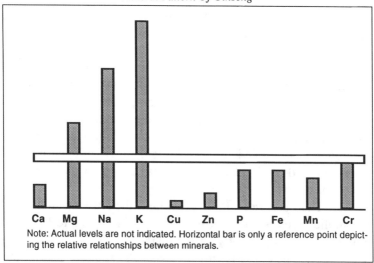

Note: Actual levels are not indicated. Horizontal bar is only a reference point depicting the relative relationships between minerals.

Figure 15
Mineral Pattern Of Comfrey

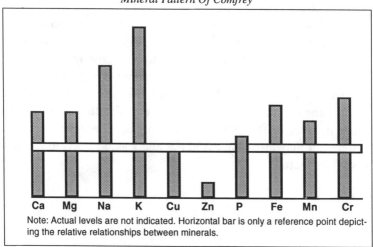

Note: Actual levels are not indicated. Horizontal bar is only a reference point depicting the relative relationships between minerals.

Drugs

Many drugs are used to sedate or stimulate the body in various ways. For example, a beta blocking drug is considered to be sedative and is intended to decrease sympathetic stimulation.

They are commonly used in the treatment of hypertension and migraine headaches.

Other drugs are used to stimulate the metabolic rate. For example, amphetamines have long been used to help control weight. Other stimulants include ephedrine, epinephrine, and tyramine.

Drugs can also interfere with nutrient absorption and utilization. For example, antacids, laxatives, anti-convulsants, corticosteroids, and anti-bacterial agents can produce a deficiency of sedative nutrients such as calcium and vitamin D. These drugs exert a chelating or leeching effect upon calcium and block the metabolic effects of vitamin D. Prolonged use of such medications can lead to rickets, osteomalacia, and other calcium deficiency disorders.

The classification of drugs and their use in individual metabolic types is a huge task in itself. This is due to the great number of drugs presently on the market as well as those being added daily. The above is only a very small example of how their use can be made more specific when metabolic types are considered. Their existence also helps to lend more credence to the fact that metabolic types exist.

Studies have shown that response to medications varies considerably from person to person. Two people can have the same health problem, but do not respond to the same medication. In fact, an individual's nutritional status can in turn affect the action and metabolism of drugs. In the future, the use of TMA may help pioneer the matching of the appropriate medication to the appropriate individual. This would aid not only in better response of the patient but may also help avoid the many side-effects associated with drug therapy.

References

Williams, R. **Biochemical Individuality.** Wiley and Sons, Pub., 1977.
Body Type Affects Uterus Cancer Risk. **J.A.M.A.** 1991.
Chengappa, K.N., et al: Handedness and Autoantibodies. **Lancet,** Sept. 14, 1991.
Sensbaugh, G.F: Biochemical Markers of Individuality. **Forensic Science Handbook.** Saferstein, R., Ed. Prentice Hall, N.J. 1982.
Watts, D.L., Heise, T.N: **Balancing Body Chemistry.** T.E.I., Dallas, TX. 1989.
Page, M: **Degeneration Regeneration.** Fla. Nutr. Dev. St. Petersburg, 1949.
Page, M: **Body Chemistry in Health and Disease.** Fla. Nutr. Dev. St.Petersburg.
Watson, G: **Nutrition And Your Mind.** Harper and Row, N.Y., 1972.
Brown, and Crounse: **Hair, Trace Elements And Human Illness.** Prager Pub., N.Y. 1980.
Hoops, H.C: The Biological Bases For Using Hair and Nails for Analysis of Trace Elements. **Trace Substances In Environmental Health VIII.** Hemphill, Ed. Conf. Univ. Mo. 1974.
Watts, D.L: Determining Osteoporotic Tendencies From Tissue Minerals Analysis of Human Hair, Type I and Type II. **Townsend Let. for Drs.** 40-41, 1986.
Watts, D.L: Water and Health. **The Newsletter.** T.E.I., Dallas, Tx. 1986.
Roe, D.A: **Drug Induced Nutritional Deficiencies.** AVI Pub., Conn. 1980.
Becking, G.C., Morrison, A.B: Hepatic Drug Metabolism in Zinc Deficient Rats. **Biochem. Pharmacol.** 19, 1970.
Dingell, J.V., Joiner, P.D., Hurwitz, L: Impairment of Drug Metabolism in Calcium Deficiency. **Biochem. Pharmacol.** 15, 1966.
Catz, C.S., et al: Effects of Iron, Riboflavin and Iodide Deficiencies on Hepatic Drug Metabolizing Systems. **J. Pharmacol. Exp. Ther.** 174, 1970.

Chapter 5

Calcium

Calcium is closely associated with the bones and teeth. In fact, 90 percent of our calcium is found in these areas. The skeleton serves as a structural support, but is actually a dynamic system. It is constantly changing and remodeling to meet mechanical needs. The skeleton changes throughout life, maximizing strength and minimizing its mass. It protects vital organs and contains much of our blood-producing tissue. In addition to these functions, the bones serve as a reservoir for calcium and other nutrients. When there is a deficiency of these nutrients, especially calcium and phosphorus, the bones are called upon to supply them to other parts of the body.

The importance of calcium in other body processes was discovered at the turn of the century when it was realized that calcium was essential in triggering heart muscle contractions. Today we know that calcium also acts as a messenger. Entering the cells through special calcium channels, calcium carries signals that initiate specific activities within the cells. Calcium influences cell division and differentiation, and helps to control the normal blood clotting mechanisms, acid-alkaline balance, and nerve conduction. Calcium also helps control endocrine secretions and is necessary to open the secretory ability of these glands, causing them to release their hormones. For example, the pancreas can release insulin only when an adequate amount of calcium is available. More recent research is showing that calcium may protect against the development of colon cancer, and alleviate high blood pressure.

The recommended daily allowance for calcium is 800 milligrams for persons over the age of 24. During pregnancy and breast feeding the requirement is 1200 milligrams. This amount is also recommended between the age of 11 to 24 years. Infants and children require 600 - 800 milligrams per day.

Calcium Regulation

Calcium is regulated by vitamin D, calcitonin, and parathyroid hormone. Calcitonin is a hormone produced by the thyroid gland, and the parathyroid hormone, or (PTH), is produced by the parathyroid gland. Vitamin D, PTH, and calcitonin influence the absorption of both calcium and phosphate from the intestinal tract, and also affect the kidneys' ability to regulate these minerals. They also regulate blood calcium and phosphate by initiating resorption of these minerals from the bone.

The hormone insulin also affects calcium, causing it to be retained by the body through reabsorption by the kidneys. Estrogen is another hormone that decreases calcium excretion. These hormones affect calcium by stimulating vitamin D activity.

The thyroid and adrenal glands can also affect calcium status. If they become overactive, they will cause the body to lose calcium. Over production of these hormones can block the effects of vitamin D, and in turn, causes poor calcium absorption from the intestines.

There are many medications that interfere with calcium absorption. Some of the most common are drugs that combat convulsion, such as phenobarbital. Antacids containing aluminum hydroxide prevent the absorption of calcium from the intestinal tract. Cortisone, which is used for the control of pain and inflammation, can contribute to a severe calcium loss with prolonged use.

Even commonly eaten foods such as rhubarb, spinach, chard, beet greens, grains, and cereals, can adversely affect one's calcium absorption. These foods contain oxalic and phytic acids, that can bind with calcium in the digestive tract, thereby decreasing absorption.

Health conditions such as malabsorption diseases that cause diarrhea can impair calcium absorption. Gastrointestinal surgeries, kidney disease, diabetes, and alcoholism can also lead to poor calcium status.

Osteoporosis

The American public has become very aware of this deleterious condition. Osteoporosis is the most widely recognized disease connected with the mineral calcium and affects over 15 million people in the U.S. alone. This condition is characterized by a loss of calcium and phosphorus from the bones, making them more porous and brittle. In this weakened condition, they are more susceptible to breaks and fractures.

One question that people often ask is, "I'm growing older, so should I take extra amounts of calcium and vitamin D to prevent osteoporosis?" The correct answer is, "Only if your individual metabolism requires it." The fact is, calcium deficiency is associated with osteoporosis, but osteoporosis can be caused by many things other than calcium deficiency. Too much calcium as well as too little calcium can cause bones to become fragile. A recent study by the Mayo Clinic reported that extra calcium supplementation tripled the risk of non-spinal fractures in some women already suffering from osteoporosis. The extra calcium intake did increase bone density all right, but the cortex of the bone was thinner and hence more fragile than normal. Some societies consume very little calcium rich products such as dairy foods and yet are not stricken with osteoporosis. A Cornell University study discovered that countries with high calcium intakes, like ours, are the ones struggling with the problem of brittle bones. Therefore, drinking three glasses of milk a day and eating plenty of dairy products can be robbing the bones of needed nutrients.

There are several reasons for this phenomenon. There are actually over 30 different mechanisms that can create fragile bones, some of which are associated with the disease process. Senile osteoporosis is a term applied mostly to men and is associated with adrenapause or adrenal insufficiency. This is due to a lack of anabolic hormone production from the adrenal glands. Adrenal hyperactivity, such as Cushings' disease, also causes osteoporosis. In this condition excessive adrenal cortical hormones cause a protein breakdown and therefore a loss of the normal protein matrix of the bone. Hyperthyroidism causes increased calcium losses and increased calcium resorption from the bone. Hyperparathyroid activity also increases calcium bone loss. Estrogen deficiency is related to bone loss, and is commonly referred to as post menopausal osteoporosis. A lack of estrogen apparently allows increased bone resorption. Too much estrogen, on the other hand, may also adversely affect bone resorption due to its relationship with other nutrients and hormones.

Immobilization due to prolonged bed rest can cause the bones to lose minerals. During space flights there is a considerable loss of bone mass in astronauts experiencing long periods of weightlessness.

A host of nutritional factors must come together to launch the brittling process. For instance, too much calcium can cause osteoporosis in tissues lacking magnesium, phosphorus, zinc, and copper. Typically, the body deposits magnesium on the surface of the bones and, if a person has a magnesium deficiency, too much calcium will exacerbate the magnesium problem. A magnesium deficiency will produce thinning of the bone cortex, making them more susceptible to breaks. Excessive amounts of vitamin D can also adversely affect the integrity of the skeleton. Nutrients that are known to be antagonistic to calcium are shown in figures 16 and 17.

Figure 16
Minerals Antagonistic To Calcium

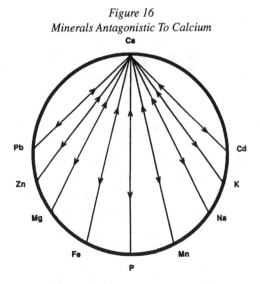

Figure 17
Vitamins Antagonistic To Calcium

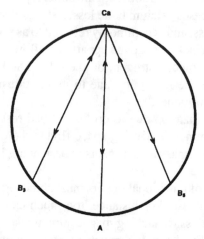

The vitamins affect calcium in a variety of ways. Vitamin A, for example, antagonizes vitamin D, and indirectly affects calcium absorption. Some vitamins stimulate the metabolic rate. This too can contribute to calcium losses or increased calcium requirements.

Type I Osteoporosis

Osteoporosis can actually be classified into two categories. Type I osteoporosis is found in people with high metabolic rates. This type is associated with thinning of the cortex, or outer portion of the bone. The body partially loses its ability to absorb and retain calcium and magnesium, causing a deficiency of these nutrients. The thyroid and adrenal glands, which are overactive in this metabolic type, produce a marked loss of calcium from the body, with an increase in phosphate retention. Activity of the parathyroid gland then slows down, rendering cells that normally produce hard bone, called osteoblasts, to become inactive.

Calcium supplements are required in this type of condition, but it may not be enough to solve the problem. In addition, the individual may need more magnesium and vitamin D, which helps to increase parathyroid hormone production. Vitamin C, copper, and zinc must also be present in adequate amounts for the ossification process to proceed.

Type II Osteoporosis

Individuals with slow metabolism suffer from type II osteoporosis. In this case, the parathyroid works overtime, increasing calcium absorption and retention, while decreasing phosphorus absorption and retention. However, this overactivity removes calcium from the medullary, or central portion of the bone. The overactive parathyroid causes a rapid increase in the number of cells that break down bones, called osteoclasts. This allows calcium to be drawn from the bone, thereby weakening it.

Since the calcium being absorbed cannot be put into the bones, the body then deposits the extra calcium in the soft tissues. This process causes calcium deposition that can result in gall stones, kidney stones, stiffness in the joints, dry skin, and premature aging and wrinkling of the skin. In this case calcium and vitamin D supplements will not solve the problem. The solution is to correct the underlying metabolic and endocrine imbalance. Once the parathyroid gland is working properly, a physician can start treating the bone problem.

In some cases, calcium bone loss can be a secondary response to an underlying metabolic problem. For example, a patient developing adult onset diabetes will suddenly have an increased need for insulin. The body will accomplish this feat by increasing parathyroid activity. This, in turn, will increase the formation of active vitamin D and cause the body to dissolve and assimilate more calcium from the skeleton. As mentioned previously, the body needs some of this extra calcium for its stepped up production and release of insulin. The extra calcium not used for this purpose can become deposited in places it's not supposed to be. Again, the diabetic condition will need to be addressed before the osteoporosis problem can be corrected. It is almost impossible to regulate the calcium level until the diabetes is under control.

When the parathyroid gland steps up its activity, the thyroid gland slows down to low gear. When this happens, patients who develop osteoporosis need to beef up the activity of their thyroids. This increased thyroid activity will slow down their overactive parathyroid glands. Conversely, if the osteoporosis is caused by an overactive thyroid coupled with increased adrenal activity, the patient will do better if the parathyroid gland gets some help.

Since osteoporosis can be caused by too much as well as too little calcium, tissue mineral analysis can be very helpful in drafting a solution to the problem. It can be used to track a host of nutrient relationships, which can clearly point a finger at the culprit causing the problem. Because there are so many contributing factors to this disease, a TMA can help develop a wholistic approach to its treatment by focusing on the body's entire biochemistry.

Factors Associated With Too Little Tissue Calcium

A shortage of calcium can cause a host of problems. Osteoporosis is the most notable, but it's not the only one. Other problems associated with a low tissue calcium include anxiety. When tissue calcium levels are low, there can be a corresponding increase in lactic acid production. The combination of these two factors can contribute to anxiety symptoms. Low calcium is related to an increased metabolic rate and hypersensitivity or irritability. It is no surprise that we find hyperactive children having low tissue calcium levels. Anything that can further lower calcium could therefore exaggerate a problem of hyperactivity. For example, grains and cereals contain phytic acid that can inhibit calcium absorption and thereby contribute to hyperactive episodes in susceptible children. Allergies are frequently found in individuals with low tissue calcium, particularly histamine allergies. Allergies also can flare up with the intake of certain foods known to interfere with calcium absorption. High blood pressure often responds to calcium supplementation. It is not unusual to find low tissue calcium in individuals with hypertension. The reason that calcium helps in controlling blood pressure is due to the sodium antagonizing effect of calcium. People who retain too much sodium frequently have a low calcium intake. Low calcium is also found in individuals suffering from rheumatoid arthritis. Insomnia has been associated with calcium for ages. Taking a warm glass of milk before bed time has been a remedy for insomnia for hundreds of years. This would certainly be helpful in individuals with a fast metabolic rate. Insomnia associated with an inability to fall asleep readily is associated with low tissue calcium. Muscle cramps, particularly those that occur at night without any real exertion, is associated with increased calcium needs.

Calcium Supplements And Depression

Serious psychological problems can arise with the extended use of calcium supplements. Dr. Richard Malter, a clinical psychologist and Director of the Malter Institute for Natural Development, in Schaumburg, Illinois, has reported a number of adverse conditions associated with calcium supplementation. Symptoms include fatigue, exhaustion, depression, anxiety, panic attacks, headaches, paranoid feelings, loss of memory and concentration, headaches, and insomnia.

One patient, who had just celebrated her fortieth birthday, read in her local newspaper about the dangers of osteoporosis attacking women her age. She began to self-medicate with calcium supplements. Soon thereafter she became depressed. Months later she was engulfed in waves of depression, coupled with fits of anger and crying spells for no apparent reason, and even became suicidal. After attending a lecture by the doctor, she put two and two together and realized that her problem began after starting the calcium supplements. She consulted with Dr. Malter, who advised that she obtain a TMA. In the meantime he suggested that she discontinue calcium supplementation. Within a very short time the anxiety attacks disappeared, the depression lifted and her mental health returned. It should be noted that the TMA confirmed that this patient should not have been taking calcium supplements at that time.

Another doctor visited us at our laboratory recently. His visit was stimulated by an article that I had written regarding the side effects of calcium and vitamin D supplements. He related that he was treating a female patient who had been suffering from severe depression for several years and who was not responding to his therapy. After reading the article, he decided to ask the patient if she was taking calcium supplements. He discovered that she had been taking very large amounts of calcium for over four years. After discussing the possibilities with her, he suggested that she discontinue the calcium. Within two weeks she was showing marked improvement.

Both women were slow metabolic types, as are 80 percent of the American population. Individuals with slow metabolism are more likely to develop these psychological problems when they take calcium supplements than fast metabolizers. Slow metabolizers require a much different approach to correcting their calcium disorder.

Dr. Malter feels that health care providers should be aware that a number of psychological problems presented by many women today may be triggered or exacerbated by calcium supplementation. This awareness may have a profound effect on the understanding and treatment of these women.

Other Factors Associated With Too Much Tissue Calcium

We frequently find that individuals who have too much tissue calcium accumulation are very susceptible to viral infections. Viruses are estimated to cause 75 percent of the body's infections, rendering these people particularly vulnerable to illness. This vulnerability may be directly related to the overabundance of calcium. Research has shown that when calcium is added to tissues containing dormant viruses, the virus will become more active and proliferate readily. The exact mechanism behind viral latency or replication is not totally known. However, a group of researchers explored this phenomenon in relation to the Epstein Barr virus (EBV). Their findings were reported in SCIENCE in 1986. Essentially, they found that when dormant EBV cells were exposed to calcium, they became active and proliferated. Blocking calcium on the other hand, prevented activation of the virus.

Viruses often produce symptoms of depression and fatigue, two signs of too much calcium. The Epstein Barr and cytomegleo viruses have been found to be associated with the chronic fatigue syndrome. Both calcium and viruses suppress the energy producing glands, the thyroid and adrenals. It is probably not a coincidence that the incidence of the chronic fatigue syndrome and associated viral conditions have risen simultaneously with increased calcium supplementation over the last several years.

Viruses may also be instrumental in triggering adult onset diabetes. Insulin release requires calcium, and it is often noted that patients with adult onset diabetes have high tissue calcium levels.

Individuals with excessive calcium, especially relative to magnesium, tend to have muscle aches and pains. A calcium-to-magnesium imbalance puts muscles in a constant state of contraction. This is especially noted in the urinary bladder. When excess calcium settles in the muscles surrounding the bladder, it will reduce the bladder's holding capacity. This will result in an increase in the frequency and urgency of urination. High tissue calcium is also associated with constipation and flatulence.

Low thyroid activity and adrenal insufficiency are commonly found in individuals with elevated tissue calcium levels. Calcium, being a sedative mineral, slows the metabolic rate. Conversely, a slowed metabolic rate allows increased tissue calcium accumulation. Excess calcium is therefore associated with fatigue and low blood pressure.

Blood Calcium

Calcium circulating in the blood should not be confused with tissue calcium. The body's tissue calcium balance is not always associated with abnormalities in the serum calcium. Deficiencies or excesses found in the tissues and blood do not always appear in tandem. A person can have too much calcium in the tissues and too little in the blood and vice-versa.

Hypocalcemia

Low blood calcium, or hypocalcemia, is a relatively rare clinical problem. It occurs when the total serum calcium falls below 7 milligrams percent. Chronic renal failure, intestinal malabsorption problems, and an inactive parathyroid gland are usually associated with this problem.

The nervous system is particularly sensitive to a low calcium level in the blood. When circulating calcium falls below a certain threshold, hyperirritability can ensue. The condition can eventually lead to sensory disturbances and dangerous heart dysfunctions. Another danger is tetany, a condition that causes periodic and painful muscular cramps and even seizures. If the condition becomes severe, the sufferer can die due to respiratory failure.

Hypercalcemia

This condition is defined as having a serum calcium above 10.5 milligrams percent. However, symptoms of the condition may not appear until the serum calcium reaches 12 milligrams. Malignancies and endocrine disorders, such as overactivity of the parathyroid gland are the chief causes of high blood calcium, or hypercalcemia. Patients who are immobilized for a long period of time can develop hypercalcemia. If the body becomes super sensitive to vitamin D, the blood will accumulate calcium. Conditions such as Paget's and Addison's diseases are associated with hypercalcemia, as well as the use of diuretic medications.

Hyperparathyroidism not only causes the blood calcium to elevate, but also causes calcium to deposit into soft tissues of the body. Symptoms of hyperparathyroidism include excessive thirst, muscle aches, recent memory loss, tendinitis, calcification of cartilage, depression, fatigue, hearing difficulties, restless legs, constipation, dyspepsia, kidney stones, gallstones, and conjunctivitis. Individuals who suffer from overactivity of the parathyroid gland have been described as having a history of bones, groans, and stones. It has also been found that when the parathyroid is working too hard, certain muscle groups lose their tone and strength. The biceps, deltoids, gluteus medius, psoas, and hamstrings are the muscles usually involved.

Vitamin-Mineral Synergists

The following vitamins and minerals are considered synergistic to calcium. These are important to know since they can improve the body's utilization of calcium. For example, even though phosphorus is antagonistic to calcium, both work together in the form of hydroxyapitite for deposition and formation of bone. Copper is necessary for the retention of calcium after it reaches the bone.

Vitamin D aids in calcium absorption, and vitamin C is involved in the formation of collagen, which is a constituent of bone matrix. This matrix has to be present for calcium to be properly deposited.

MINERALS SYNERGISTIC TO CALCIUM	
Magnesium	Phosphorus
Copper	Sodium
Potassium	Selenium

VITAMINS SYNERGISTIC TO CALCIUM	
Vitamin D	Vitamin E
Vitamin C	Vitamin A

Conclusion

As with most minerals, calcium is best evaluated in relationship to its other co-factors, whether it is tested through blood, tissue or excretion studies. When the synergistic and antagonistic nutrients are taken into consideration, fewer conflicting and more fruitful results may be forthcoming with the nutritional treatment of disorders associated with calcium, particularly osteoporosis. Many diseases may precipitate bone loss, and osteoporosis may be a secondary problem. Treating the whole person instead of a disease, or single nutrient imbalance, may also prove more rewarding and beneficial to many of those afflicted with osteoporosis. Osteoporosis should be considered a metabolic defect rather than a simple calcium deficiency. As we can see from the calcium mineral and vitamin wheels, there is a lot more to consider than calcium alone.

References

Garland, F., et al. Can colon cancer incidence and death rates be reduced with calcium and vitamin D? **Am. J. Clin. Nutr.** 54,193S-201S, 1991

Wargovich, M.J., et al. Modulation effects of calcium in animal models of colon carcinogenesis and short-term studies in subjects at increased risk for colon cancer. **Am. J. Clin. Nutr.** 54,202S-205S, 1991

Nordin, C., et al: The problem of calcium requirement. **Am. J. Clin. Nutr.** 45,5, 1987.

Berridge, M.J: The interaction of cyclic nucleotides and calcium in the control of cellular activity. **Advances in Cyclic Nucleotide Research,** Vol. 6. Greengard, P., Robison, G.A., Eds. Raven Press, N.Y., 1975.

Monnier, L., et al: Intestinal and renal handling of calcium in human diabetes mellitus: Influence of acute oral glucose loading and diabetic control. **J. Clin. Invest.** 8, 1978.

Recker, R.R., et al: Effects of estrogens and calcium carbonates on bone loss in post-menopausal women. **Ann. Int. Med.** 87, 1977.

Aub, J.C., et al: Studies of calcium and phosphorus metabolism III. The effects of thyroid hormones and thyroid disease. **J. Clin. Invest.** 7, 1929.

Krane, S.M., et al: The effects of thyroid disease in calcium metabolism in man. **J. Clin. Invest.** 35, 1956.

Kleeman, C.B., et al: Metabolic observation in a case of thyrotoxicosis with hypercalcuria. **J. Clin. Invest.** 18, 1958.

Harrison, H.E., Harrison, H.C: Transfer of calcium across intestinal wall in relation to action of vitamin D and cortisol. **Am. J. Physiol.** 99, 1960.

Massry, S.G: Renal handling of calcium. **Disorders of Mineral Metabolism.** Vol.II. Bronner, R., Coburn, J., Eds. Academic Press, N.Y., 1982.

Shafer, R.B., Nuttal, F.Q: Calcium and folic acid absorption in patients taking anticonvulsant drugs. **Metab. Clin. Exp.** 41, 1975.

O'Donovan, D.K: The diagnosis of latent tetany, with observations on the effect of calciferol. **Brit. Med. J.** 2, 1948.

Sholz, D.A., et al: Diagnostic considerations in hypercalcemic syndromes. **Medical Clinics of North America,** 56, 1972.

Jorgenson, H: Hypercalcemia in adrenal-cortical insufficiency. **Acta. Med. Scand.** 193, 1973.

Lowe, C.E., Bird, E.D., Thomas, W.C: Hypercalcemia in myxedema. **J. Clin. Endocrin. Metab.** 22, 1962.
Baxter, J.D., Bondy, P.K: Hypercalcemia of thyrotoxicosis. **Ann. Int. Med.** 65, 1966.
Parfitt, A.M: Chlorothiazide-induced hypercalcemia in juvenile osteoporosis and hyperparathyroidism. **N.E.J.M.** 281, 1969.
Micher, W.C., et al: Primary hyperparathyroidism. **Arch. Int. Med.** 107, 1961.
McCarron, D.A: Calcium and magnesium nutrition in human hypertension. **Ann. Int. Med.** 98,5, 1983.
Lasaridis, D.A., et al: Calcium diet supplementation increased urinary sodium excretion in essential hypertension. **Nephron.** 45, 1987.
Harrison, M., Fraser, R., Mullan, B: Calcium metabolism in osteoporosis: Acute and long-term responses to increased calcium intake. **Lancet,** 1961.
Schwartz, E., Panariello, A., Saeli, J: Radioactive calcium kinetics during high calcium intake in osteoporosis. **J. Clin. Invest.** 44, 1965.
Riis, B., et al: Does calcium supplementation prevent post menopausal bone loss? **N.E.J.M.** 316, 1987.
Adams, P., et al: Parathyroid function in spontaneous primary hypothyroidism. **J. Endocrinol.** 40, 1968.
Bouillon, R., DeMoor, P: Parathyroid function in patients with hyper-or hypothyroidism. **J. Clin. Endocrinol.** 38, 1974.
Bortz, W., et al: Differentiation between thyroid and parathyroid causes of hypercalcemia. **Ann. Int. Med.** 54, 1961.
Clark, I., Geoffroy, R.F., Bowers, W: Effects of adrenal cortical steroids on calcium metabolism. **Endocrinol.** 64, 1959.

Chapter 6

Magnesium

You just heard on the news your company is a takeover candidate. You fret about your job security. You have to give a big presentation to the largest potential client your company has ever courted. You worry about the outcome. Your spouse has decided to file for divorce. Your friends take you out for a drink after work to help you get over the shock.

Emotional stress and alcohol consumption are two of the many ways Americans lose magnesium, a critical trace element essential to physical health and well-being.

Excessive exertion such as tennis, bicycling, running, and cross country skiing are physical stresses that can tax magnesium reserves. Women who are pregnant, mothers breast feeding their infants, people on medications, or who develop frequent infections can also find themselves with a shortage of this critical mineral.

Magnesium is the fourth most abundant cation in the human body. Approximately 25 grams are present in an adult. Half of that amount is contained in the bones with the remainder found in soft tissues. The highest concentration is found in the skeletal muscles, followed by the liver, heart, and pancreas.

Magnesium is a key element in cellular metabolism. The higher the metabolic rate of a cell, the higher its magnesium requirement. The mineral is also extensively involved in vital enzyme systems throughout the body. Its positive charge triggers many enzyme reactions, of which over 300 are known. Even the important nucleic acids of the cells, DNA and RNA, are stabilized by this mineral.

Problems Created By Magnesium Deficiencies

Because magnesium is a natural sedative, the more serious the magnesium deficit, the edgier a person may become. An individual can become excessively anxious and short tempered. It's a good bet that if someone jumps at the slightest provocation, they have a magnesium shortfall. Hyper-irritability almost always results after a major magnesium loss. Adults may even suffer muscle tremors, memory loss, inability to concentrate, apathy, and depression; children can become hyperactive. Magnesium can help calm nerves and improve mental concentration in many anxiety ridden individuals.

Increased Perspiration And Body Odor

Although anxiety is a telltale sign of magnesium deficiency, there are other obvious problems. Excessive perspiration is a common trait with individuals who have a magnesium deficiency. Even the slightest amount of exertion causes them to break out in a sweat. Foul body odor is another physical sign of magnesium deficiency.

Muscle Cramps

One of magnesium's primary roles in the body is to prevent excess accumulation of calcium within cells and around joints. It is one of nature's most potent calcium blockers. People suffering from relative magnesium deficiencies can have excess calcium accumulation in tissues other than bone, leading to a wide range of conditions centering around this calcium build up. Magnesium deficiencies can leave muscles in a cramped and tense state, causing hyperactive reflexes. A muscle will contract when calcium enters the muscle cell. The appearance of calcium causes magnesium to build up in the cell. When the concentration of magnesium is high enough, calcium exits the cell. At that point the muscles relax. This delicate balance of calcium and magnesium is responsible for normal muscular activity and transmission of nerve impulses. If the magnesium concentration is not adequate however, some calcium will remain in the cell. This causes the muscle to remain in a tonic, or slightly contracted state. Not enough magnesium can cause muscle cramps with the slightest exertion. This is a common problem in athletes. The hands and feet are particularly prone to cramps at night with a magnesium deficiency.

Magnesium affects the balance between the extra cellular and intracellular fluids by influencing sodium and potassium. Normalization of potassium in the cell is very dependent upon magnesium. In the presence of magnesium, potassium is taken into the cells and sodium is pumped out. Magnesium deficiency can therefore lead to increased sodium and fluid retention.

Cardio-Vascular Conditions

Excessive calcium deposits can be dangerous to the cardiovascular system. People with a relative magnesium deficiency do not have the proper balance of calcium and magnesium in the cells to make the muscles operate correctly. They experience diastolic high blood pressure because their heart and arterial blood vessels cannot relax completely during the resting stage of the heart beat. This happens because the added amount of calcium continues to prolong the muscular contraction. Systolic hypertension, on the other hand, is a frequent finding in people with an absolute magnesium deficiency. The hypertension results from increased or intensified contraction in both the arterial and heart muscles. Research has shown that magnesium deficiency is found in individuals who suffered sudden ischemic heart attacks. This is more commonly referred to as a stress induced heart attack, and is associated with a concomitant elevation of adrenal stress hormones.

Magnesium is also helpful for sufferers of athero- and arteriosclerosis, which results from fat and calcium deposits in the arteries. Magnesium helps in relaxing the arteries and therefore controls blood pressure in many.

Conventional cardiologists are beginning to recognize the importance of this valuable nutrient in those suffering with heart disease. Recent investigations have found that magnesium deficiency is associated with hypertryglyceridemia and hypercholesterolemia. The mechanism is related to excessive production and release of lipids into the circulation along with an impaired ability for removal. Also, the low density lipoproteins (LDL), and very low density lipoproteins (VLDL) increase, and the high density lipoproteins (HDL) decrease when not enough magnesium is present. A deficiency of this mineral apparently allows a modification of lipoproteins, making them susceptible to oxidative damage, which can contribute to the athero- and arteriosclerotic process.

Arthritis-Stones-Bursitis

Osteoarthritis results from calcium deposits within the joints. When magnesium deficiency exists, excessive quantities of calcium can build up in tissues such as the tendons and ligaments. Painful bursitis is caused by the same mechanism. Gallstones and calcium phosphate kidney stones are agonizing conditions that result from an overabundance of calcium in the wrong places. Many of these conditions respond well to magnesium supplementation. When combined with vitamin B_6, magnesium works to prevent these painful accretions.

Urinary Frequency - Constipation

The same problem can affect the bladder. Since the muscles surrounding the bladder do not relax completely, it cannot hold its normal volume. Even though there is not an excess amount of urine being produced, the sufferer feels a great urgency to urinate frequently. Constipation is also frequently found in individuals with a relative deficiency of magnesium. This is due to muscular constriction, causing poor peristalsis or intestinal motility. Magnesium can be considered a natural laxative.

Toxic Shock Syndrome

Researchers discovered the toxic shock syndrome triggered by super absorbent tampons was caused, in part, by a magnesium deficiency. These tampons absorbed magnesium from the vaginal area. At the same time, a bacteria, staphylococcus aureus, proliferated. Researchers theorized staph aureus thrives more readily in the absence of magnesium.

Insomnia

Even sleep can be affected by the lack of magnesium. People who do not have enough magnesium in their systems tend to fall asleep readily. However, they only experience a relatively short period of deep restful sleep. During most of the night they are only in a light sleep. They toss and turn and often wake up exhausted. This type of insomnia develops especially when one has been under stress.

Epilepsy-Seizure Disorders-Pregnancy

Magnesium deficiency has been linked to even more deleterious effects such as convulsions, seizures, tetany and epilepsy.

Expectant mothers who suffer from pre-eclampsia often have magnesium deficiency. The lack of magnesium during pregnancy can lead to spasm of the umbilical arteries and can actually affect nutrition to the unborn fetus.

Premenstrual syndrome (PMS) and depression are other physical and emotional disorders that have been linked to a low level of magnesium.

In summary, the following conditions have been associated with magnesium deficiency in scientific literature. These conditions have also been reported to respond favorably to magnesium therapy.

CONDITIONS ASSOCIATED WITH MAGNESIUM DEFICIENCY	
Atherosclerosis	Arteriosclerosis
Arrhythmia	Myocardial Infarction
Congestive Heart Failure	Eclampsia
Osteoporosis	Chronic Fatigue Syndrome
Premenstrual Syndrome	Hormonal Imbalance
Diabetes	Immune Regulation
Lipid Disorders	Blood Sugar Disorders

Causes Of Magnesium Deficiencies

Potential trouble looms when a magnesium deficiency occurs. Unfortunately, the body has a variety of ways to develop a magnesium deficiency. A deficiency results if the body excretes more magnesium than normal, or if it cannot absorb the mineral properly. This problem is called an "absolute" deficiency. A "relative" deficiency is possible too. This occurs when the cells choose to stockpile other elements in relation to their reserves of magnesium. The net effect is a magnesium deficiency because the body's delicate mineral balance has been upset. Because the body has a host of processes that can create a net magnesium loss, each person responds differently to magnesium problems and cures.

Magnesium is particularly sensitive to stress. When some individuals are placed under mental or physical duress, their bodies increase magnesium excretion. This can exacerbate the problem because magnesium is a natural sedative. At a time when their bodies need more magnesium to weather the storm, physiological forces are eliminating the magnesium they currently have.

In addition, certain foods interfere with magnesium absorption. For example, foods that contain phytate prevent the body from using this vital mineral. Phytate is an acid that binds minerals in the intestinal tract causing them to be excreted unused. Phytates are found in grains and cereals.

Alcohol and magnesium do not mix. Alcohol hastens the excretion of magnesium through the kidneys. It is common to find severe magnesium deficiencies in alcoholics.

Clinical disorders can also be a culprit. Sprue, bowel resection, prolonged diarrhea, alcoholic cirrhosis, diabetic acidosis, pancreatitis, excessive lactation, renal disease, and malignant osteolytic bone disease all interfere with the body's proper absorption of magnesium. Individuals with intestinal disorders such as celiac disease lose large amounts of magnesium in their stools, as much as four times normal.

Certain medications interfere with magnesium retention. Diuretics particularly can cause increased magnesium excretion through the kidneys. Other drugs such as laxatives can also interfere with magnesium absorption.

The Endocrine Glands And Magnesium

The thyroid, parathyroid and adrenal glands significantly influence magnesium in the body. Increased thyroid activity speeds up the metabolic rate. The body needs increased levels of magnesium to keep pace. It is therefore common to find lowered magnesium levels in patients suffering from hyperthyroidism. The opposite is true for those with underactive thyroid glands.

The parathyroid gland also affects magnesium. Increased parathyroid activity amplifies the intestinal absorption of calcium and causes the kidney to reabsorb it. If the gland becomes overactive, a "relative" magnesium deficiency will result. However, if the parathyroid underachieves, a magnesium deficiency also results. This is because the thyroid and the parathyroid act in opposition. If one gland increases output, the other automatically decreases its hormonal production or activity. Thus, if the parathyroid lowers its secretions, thyroid activity increases, leading to lower magnesium levels.

Magnesium supplementation can help to improve both hypo and hyperparathyroid conditions. When patients suffering from hypoparathyroidism ingest magnesium, the mineral stimulates their parathyroid activity. Magnesium, on the other hand, will have a slowing down effect on an overactive parathyroid gland.

A similar scenario exists with the adrenal glands. When either the medullary or cortical portions of the adrenal glands work overtime, they trigger increased magnesium excretion. Increased magnesium intake will help to slow down this over activity.

Minerals Antagonistic To Magnesium

Magnesium requirements are affected by stress, diet and certain medications. In addition, at least twenty-eight nutritional factors impact magnesium levels. Figure 18 lists the minerals that are antagonistic to magnesium. Excessive intake or increased retention of any one or any combination of these elements can induce an absolute or relative magnesium deficiency. These antagonisms can occur on both absorptive and metabolic levels.

Toxic metals such as lead interfere with most nutrient minerals, including magnesium. Adequate amounts of magnesium in the diet, or magnesium supplementation can greatly reduce lead absorption from the intestinal tract. Antagonism between lead and magnesium also occurs on a metabolic level, since lead accumulates in the mitochondrial membrane of cells, an area where magnesium is most needed.

Cadmium, another toxic metal, can also cause problems when an excessive amount accumulates in the body. This build up will stimulate portions of the adrenal cortex, which results in a magnesium loss. This loss, in turn, leads to an increased retention of sodium, which can then contribute to high blood pressure. Magnesium supplementation can help prevent and control cadmium-induced high blood pressure.

The balance between calcium and magnesium controls the release of many of the body's hormones. For example, the pancreas requires calcium to be able to release insulin. Physicians have discovered increased levels of tissue calcium relative to magnesium in individuals who produce higher than normal amounts of insulin. This condition causes hypoglycemia or low blood sugar. Conversely, those with elevated magnesium levels relative to calcium do not release enough insulin which contributes to high blood sugar or hyperglycemia.

Both manganese and iron decrease the absorption of magnesium directly. However, manganese can substitute for magnesium in some enzyme systems.

Figure 18
Minerals Antagonistic To Magnesium

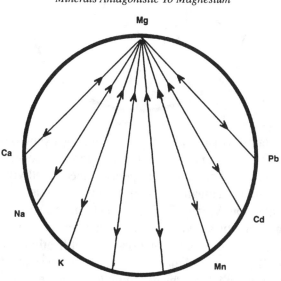

The minerals shown in Figure 18, are mutually antagonistic to magnesium. Be aware that magnesium in the appropriate amounts can also beneficially antagonize the toxic metals. But, if these nutritional minerals or toxic metals become excessive, they can in turn produce a deficiency of magnesium as well.

Vitamins Antagonistic To Magnesium

Vitamins can antagonize magnesium by increasing magnesium's metabolic requirements. Figure 19 shows the vitamins that are considered antagonistic to magnesium.

Figure 19
Vitamins Antagonistic To Magnesium

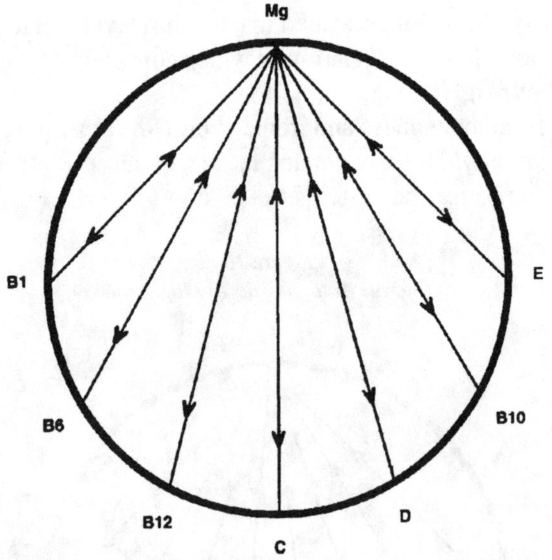

Vitamin D can indirectly cause a magnesium deficiency by increasing calcium absorption, which in turn stresses magnesium reserves. Vitamin D also triggers elevated parathyroid activity, which leads to a magnesium deficiency, again due to increased calcium retention. Vitamin B_1, C, E, and B_6 have a stimulating effect upon metabolic activity, which increases magnesium requirements in cellular enzymatic functions. The utilization of thiamin, or vitamin B_1, requires adequate amounts of magnesium. Thiamin cannot be utilized when a magnesium deficiency exists. In addition, when thiamin is given to a person with a low magnesium, it can aggravate the magnesium deficiency.

Large doses of vitamin E can occasionally cause hypertensive effects in some people. This effect is caused by too little magnesium.

Vitamin B_{12} contains the element cobalt, which can cause cardiac problems when present in excess. In the 1940's, beer companies added cobalt to beer to enhance the foam formation. Heavy beer drinkers began to experience heart problems that were found to be caused by magnesium deficiency. The deficiency was exacerbated by the excessive cobalt intake. Chromium is now used to augment the foam formation in beers. Folic acid increases the activity of a number of glycolytic enzymes requiring magnesium. This stepped up activity can increase the body's metabolic need for magnesium.

Vitamin-Mineral Synergists

The following minerals and vitamins are synergistic to magnesium.

MINERALS SYNERGISTIC TO MAGNESIUM		
Calcium	Chromium	Manganese
Phosphorus	Potassium	Zinc

VITAMINS SYNERGISTIC TO MAGNESIUM		
Vitamin A	Vitamin B_1	Vitamin B_2
Vitamin B_3	Vitamin C	Vitamin E

Synergistic nutrients enhance the absorption and the metabolic utilization of magnesium. In the body, events rarely happen in a vacuum. This is why some people do not respond to magnesium supplements regardless of the dosage. Increasing the amount of magnesium significantly above the RDA will not help. This is because the other nutrients required to solve the problem are not present in their proper proportions. When the difficulty is viewed as a whole and all the nutrients are available in an appropriate balance, beneficial results will happen often at relatively small doses.

Maintaining mineral content in the body is like walking a tight rope. Remember, single deficiencies rarely develop alone. Typically a deficiency of a synergistic nutrient will develop also. This explains why some vitamins and minerals can be both beneficial and detrimental. Within a narrow physiological range, a nutrient can act synergistically. However, when a nutrient becomes concentrated in the body in higher, more dangerous amounts, it can block absorption of another nutrient or increase its requirements in metabolic functions.

Because magnesium is so important to proper body functioning, its Recommended Dietary Allowances (RDA) are fairly high. Here are the suggested amounts:

Infants	40 to 70 milligrams
Children	50 to 250 milligrams
Adults	300 to 400 milligrams
Pregnant or lactating mothers:	450 milligrams

Foods that are high in magnesium include nuts and green leafy vegetables. Magnesium is a constituent of chlorophyll in green plants.

Conclusion

The role of magnesium in important biological processes is extensive. Recognition of both its synergistic and antagonistic roles with other nutrients can greatly enhance its therapeutic effectiveness, thus avoiding nutritionally induced deficiencies.

As with other minerals, the blood will always maintain normalcy at the expense of tissue stores of magnesium. Tissue mineral analysis of the hair is one of the most valuable laboratory tools for evaluating magnesium status when assessed according to its physiological range with other nutritional factors.

References

Seelig, M.S: **Magnesium Deficiency in the Pathogenesis of Disease.** Plenum Pub., N.Y. 1980.
Richardson, J.A., Welt, L.G: Hypomagnesemia of Vitamin D Administration. **Proc. Soc. Exper. Biol. & Med.** 118, 1965.
Fourman, P., Morgan, D.B: Chronic Magnesium Deficiency. **Proc. Nutr. Soc.** 21, 1962.
MacIntyre, I., et al: Intracellular Magnesium Deficiency in Man. **Clin. Sci.** 20, 1961.
Theodore, H., Siddiqui, D.A: Magnesium and the Pancreas. **Am. J. Clin. Nutr.** 26, 1973.
Ramsay, I: **Thyroid Disease and Muscle Function.** Yearbook Pub., Inc., Chicago, Ill. 1974.
Jones, J.E., et al: Magnesium Metabolism in Hyperthyroidism and Hypothyroidism. **J. Clin. Invest.** 45, 1966.
Doe, R.P., et al: Magnesium Metabolism in Hyperthyroidism. **J. Lab. & Clin. Med.** 54, 1959.
Jones, K.H., Fourman, P: Effects of infusion of Magnesium and of Calcium in Parathyroid insufficiency. **Clin. Sci.** 30, 1966.
Homer, L: Hypoparathyroidism Requiring Massive Amounts of Medication, with Apparent Responses to Magnesium Sulfate. **J. Clin. Endocrinol. & Metab.** 21, 1961.
Hanna, S. MacIntyre, I: Influence of Aldosterone on Magnesium Metabolism. **Lancet** 2, 1960.
Wacker, W.E., Vallee, B.L: Magnesium Metabolism. **N.E.J.M.** 254, 1958.
Fine, B.P: Influence of Magnesium on the Intestinal Absorption of Lead. **Environ. Res.** 12, 1976.
Malaisse, W.J., et al: The Stimulus-Secretion Coupling of Glucose-Induced Insulin Release. **J. Lab. Clin. Med.** 76, 1970.
Bennett, L.L., et al: Calcium-Magnesium Antagonism in Insulin Secretion by the Perfused Rat Pancreas. **Endocrinol.** 85, 1969.
Leclercqu-Meyer, V., et al: Effect of Calcium and Magnesium on Glucagon Secretion. **Endocrinol.** 93, 1973.
Itokawa, Y., Fujiwara, M: Changes in tissue magnesium, calcium and phosphorus levels in magnesium deficient rats in relation to thiamin excess and deficiency. **J. Nutr.** 103, 1973.
Watts, D.L: The Assessment of Hypertensive Tendencies from Hair Trace Element Analysis. **Chiro. Econ.** Mar., 1986.
Brisco, A.M., Regan, C: Effects of Magnesium on Calcium Metabolism in Man. **Am. J. Clin. Nutr.** 19, 1966.
Epidemic Cardiac Failure in Beer Drinkers. **Nutr. Rev.** 26, 1968.
Alexander, C.S: Cobalt-Beer Cardiomyopathy. **Am. J. Med.** 53, 1972.

Chapter 7

Copper

Ever wonder why some people with arthritis swear that their pain is helped when wearing a copper bracelet? Or why some people have been taking iron for years and can't seem to improve their iron poor blood? Why women that are on the verge of menstruation are more likely to catch a cold or flu? Why frontal headaches occur in women when nearing their monthly cycle, or why they develop cravings for things such as chocolate, avocados, and white wine? Why people develop a form of color blindness causing them to have difficulty distinguishing certain shades of green and blue? Why people become moody or depressed after eating certain foods? The answers to these questions may center around the amount of copper in their bodies.

Conditions Associated With Copper Deficiency

The ideal copper content of a healthy adult is approximately eighty milligrams. The highest level of copper is found in the liver and brain, followed by the heart, kidneys, pancreas, spleen, lungs, bones, and muscles. Copper is an essential constituent of many important cellular enzymes such as, cytochrome c oxidase, superoxide dismutase, dopamine B-hydroxylase, lysyl oxidase, tyrosinase, and monoamine oxidase. A deficiency or excess of copper can disrupt the function of these important enzymes.

Copper And Anemia

One of the earliest conditions found to be associated with copper deficiency was anemia. When a copper deficiency is present, the body has difficulty utilizing iron properly. For instance, when red blood cells age and are broken down, their iron content is sequestered. Normally this iron is eventually incorporated into new red blood cells that carry oxygen to the cells of the body. If a copper deficiency is present, this iron, as well as iron taken in from the diet, cannot be properly utilized by the red blood cells. Iron will then build up in storage areas throughout the body. Anemia eventually develops even in the face of adequate iron levels in the body. This condition cannot be corrected by adding more iron to the diet. Instead, increased copper is required to correct this type of anemia. In fact, a deficiency of copper can actually cause excessive iron build-up and contribute to a host of health conditions.

Copper And Arthritis

As mentioned previously, when a copper deficiency occurs, iron builds up in the tissues because the body cannot employ it properly. Often, the excess iron is deposited in the joints, contributing to rheumatoid arthritis. Studies have shown that this type of arthritis becomes much more severe in animals on a copper deficient diet. One study found that the tissue iron content was over 400 percent above normal during the experimental copper deficient diet.

TMA studies of patients with rheumatoid arthritis frequently show a low tissue copper level. Chronic cases often show a high iron-to-copper ratio. There are factors that can contribute to the development of this condition other than low dietary copper, or high dietary iron. A chronic bacterial infection can cause this imbalance between iron and copper. This is why rheumatoid arthritis can develop following an infectious disease. The infection can cause a depletion of the body's copper stores, thereby allowing iron accumulation in the joints.

It is well known that patients enjoy a spontaneous relief of arthritis when they contract a condition that causes an increase in copper retention. For example, pregnancy and gall bladder obstruction cause an increase in copper retention. Many women have reported improvement in their arthritic symptoms when they become pregnant. As copper levels normally rise during the course of pregnancy. Many men suffering from rheumatoid arthritis report marked relief after developing gallstones. Copper is normally excreted through the gallbladder. When the bladder is obstructed, copper excretion diminishes and can therefore build up in the body as a result.

These effects of copper explain why many sufferers of rheumatoid arthritis obtain relief when wearing copper bracelets. In some individuals the copper is absorbed through the skin, supplying the helpful element to the painful joints. A study carried out on arthritic patients in Australia has substantiated this "wives tale".

Rheumatoid arthritis apparently became more prevalent in America as the country rapidly industrialized. This industrialization created increased production of commonly used elements that are antagonistic to copper, such as cadmium, zinc, and lead. It has been recorded that Europeans before the Industrial Revolution were rarely bothered by this disease. Rainsford hypothesizes that Europeans used copper cooking and eating utensils, thus boosting their copper intake.

Osteoarthritis on the other hand is associated with tissue copper levels that are above normal. Too much copper in the body can cause calcium accumulation around the joints, causing aching and stiffness.

Bacterial Infections

Bacteria require iron for proliferation, therefore, during a bacterial infection the body sequesters iron from the blood. The iron becomes stored in the liver, spleen, bone, and lymphatic tissues during the course of the infection. At the same time, the body mobilizes copper from storage tissues. Increased copper levels in the blood allow the body to mount an effective attack and overcome the invading organism. Simply put, during a bacterial infection, the normal response is a reduction in the blood ratio of iron relative to copper. This is a normal response, but if the infection becomes chronic, tissue copper stores can become depleted, at the same time causing an excess tissue storage of iron.

TMA studies of individuals with a chronic infection usually show a high tissue iron to copper ratio. This would be the opposite of what is occurring in the blood. The most common cause of a chronic bacterial infection is due to a dental abscess. We have found individuals who have had this type of infection for several years without really knowing it.

As discussed previously, a chronic bacterial infection can result in what is termed an "infectious anemia". This is due to the chronic depletion of copper caused by the infection resulting in excess iron accumulation throughout the body tissues. This can result in chronic fatigue. Patients with this condition usually feel tired and run down. They develop lowered resistance and become susceptible to recurring infections. Normal copper levels must be restored in order for the body to use this stored iron.

Neurological Disorders

Copper, either too much or too little, can affect the central nervous system. We have found that patients who suffer from neurological disorders such as multiple sclerosis and Parkinson's disease, usually have a severe copper deficiency on their TMA tests. These observations have been reported by others. Douglas reported finding significant differences in hair copper levels in 40 multiple sclerosis patients compared to 42 control subjects. Similar findings have been observed in patients with Parkinson's disease.

Animal studies have also confirmed a copper relationship to this condition. Levels of dopamine, a neurotransmitter in the brain, were found low in copper deficient animals. Low dopamine levels are common in human patients suffering from Parkinson's disease. Copper is an essential element in dopamine metabolism.

Copper is required for the normal myelination of nerves. Myelin is a fatty substance that acts as insulation around nerves. When this insulation is missing, the material surrounding the nerves harden or sclerose. Therefore, abnormal neurological discharge results in spasticity, tremors, and paralysis.

Menkes disease, also known as Steely Hair disease, is an inherited inborn error of copper metabolism in infants. The condition is often fatal with a life expectancy of only two years. The children eventually manifest severe neurological disturbances, as well as a coarse, steely consistency of the hair. This devastating condition emphasizes the need for nutritional monitoring of the fetus. Baumslag has reported the practicality of using TMA for monitoring the copper status of the fetus through the mother. If the tissue levels of copper are low in the mother, the fetus could be provided the mineral by increasing copper in the mother's diet, or by supplementation. Copper easily crosses the placenta barrier.

Cardiovascular Disorders

Copper is a critical component for the integrity of the cardiovascular system. An adequate amount of copper is required to produce the necessary enzymes which maintain, among other things, the connective tissues. A roster of feared heart ailments — aneurysms, heart enlargement, heart failure, infarcts and ischemic heart disease—are known to result from copper deficiency.

When the body has a deficiency of copper relative to zinc, there is a decrease in the formation of high density lipoproteins (HDL), and an increase in low density lipoproteins (LDL). HDLs are the "good" molecules that help fight coronary heart disease, particularly atherosclerosis. This imbalance can lead to hardening of the arteries, regardless of the total serum cholesterol or triglyceride levels.

Too much copper in the system can also contribute to cardiovascular problems. Thyroid activity is reduced in the presence of too much copper. For many years it has been known that low thyroid activity is associated with hypercholesterolemia.

Malignancies And Copper

Low tissue copper levels are common with some malignancies, generally the catabolic or highly metastatic types. Patients suffering from Hodgkin's disease have an elevated iron-to-copper ratio, especially in their lymph nodes.

Continued cancer research is discovering that some malignancy conditions step up the body's needs for copper. Copper is a key component in normal cell functioning because it helps regulate cellular respiration. When researchers added copper to the diet of laboratory animals, the mineral noticeably decreased tumor growth and slowed its spread. These actions also increased the survival rate of the animals.

Scientists have conducted extensive research to prove that viruses cause cancer. However, there have been no conclusive findings in this area. Malignancies do develop following severe viral and bacterial infections, but in my opinion, they are not necessarily the causative agents. The resulting imbalance between copper and iron sets the stage for the biological prerequisites for cancer, creating a biochemical predisposition to the disease.

There are a number of other conditions seen through TMA studies that are associated with copper deficiency. These include gout, hypertension, antibiotic sensitivity, hyperactivity, hyperglycemia, emotional disturbances (manic disorders), insomnia, allergies and osteoporosis.

Conditions Associated With Copper Toxicity

Copper toxicity, unfortunately, is common in the United States. Copper intake is typically three to five milligrams per day. Areas that have high copper or low zinc soils tend to have populations with excessive tissue copper levels. The hardness of the area's drinking water also plays a major role in copper toxicity.

In many cases, copper water pipes are the culprit. A good indicator of copper in residential and commercial buldings is the appearance of a bluish green discoloration on porcelain plumbing fixtures. The mineral also enters the food chain because feed lots add copper to their animals' diets. Farmers also use copper to spray vegetables and grains to prevent fungus and algae growth.

Individuals metabolize copper at different rates, making copper toxicity a personal affair. The slower the metabolic rate, the higher the copper retention, regardless of copper intake. The reverse is also true, the higher the metabolic rate, the less copper accumulates. It has been found that vegetarians seem to have a greater ability to retain copper than non-vegetarians.

Increased copper retention can develop as a result of severe viral infections such as mononucleosis and hepatitis. Copper toxicity also can develop if a person does not have enough vitamin C, B_6, B_3, B_5 and A, or the minerals zinc and iron. These are nutrients antagonistic to copper, as shown in figures 22 and 23.

A dire example of what can happen to an individual with too much copper is Wilson's disease. This is an inborn error of metabolism which causes toxic amounts of copper to accumulate in the liver. Thereafter, the excess copper begins to invade other tissues, ending up in the brain. Excess copper can become deposited in the eyes, causing a copper ring to form in the cornea, a sure diagnostic sign of the disease.

Premenstrual Syndrome (PMS) And Copper

Estrogen is closely associated with copper; when the level of one rises, so does the other. Zinc is associated with progesterone; the levels of these two also move in tandem. Many women taking oral contraceptives have elevated tissue copper levels. The same is true for women using copper intrauterine devices, since the body absorbs the copper from the copper wire. Many gynecologists believe that this copper absorption is the mechanism of pregnancy prevention. An imbalance between the hormones estrogen and progesterone, as well as zinc, copper and other nutiritional factors, is likely to be the chief culprit contributing to menstrual abnormalities.

It is common to find women who suffer from PMS to have elevated tissue copper, with low tissue zinc. PMS symptoms echo the aches and pains of copper toxicity: frontal headaches, depression, fatigue, constipation, emotional volatility, weight gain, and food cravings. The symptoms vary depending on the severity of copper toxicity. They subside after the period ends, which is when progesterone and zinc levels start rising.

One way to calm PMS symptoms is to supplement the diet with zinc and vitamin B_6. If these do not work alone, they might need a little help from magnesium and other B vitamins. Typically these nutrients will help in controlling these symptoms, especially the devastating frontal headaches.

Copper levels also affect menstrual flow. If a woman has a high tissue copper level, her flow may be prolonged and heavy. However, if her zinc levels predominate, she may have a light and short menstrual flow, and her breasts may become extremely tender. Too much copper, on the other hand, can also stop menstruation. Patients with anorexia nervosa typically stop menstruating. We commonly find very high tissue copper levels in patients suffering from anorexia and bulemia.

It has been found that the zinc levels will usually rise after menstruation. If the concentration becomes too high, then zinc can contribute to a post-menstrual syndrome. Women with soaring zinc concentrations may retain water and develop feelings of anxiousness, indecisiveness, and depression. Post-menstrual syndrome is associated with low estrogen and therefore, copper supplementation may be required in women with this condition.

Toxemia And Post Partum Depression

Copper and estrogen levels normally rise during pregnancy, especially during the last trimester. When copper levels become too high, however, it can be associated with pregnancy complications, including toxemia, eclampsia, and postpartum depression.

After delivery, the mother's copper levels often returns to normal. However, many women retain their excessive copper stores long after they have delivered. The reason may be due to the development of gallstones during pregnancy. Pregnancy increases the susceptibility to gallstones several-fold and therefore results in the inability to excrete the mineral. Copper toxicity can become a real problem if pregnancies are close together. What's worse, increased copper accumulation in the mother can lead to inherited copper toxicity in the children.

Some women actually feel much better once they conceive. If this occurs, they probably had more progesterone (zinc) than estrogen (copper) in their systems before the pregnancy. Conversely, women who feel terrible while carrying a baby probably started with too much estrogen and copper coursing through their veins. The pregnancy increased those already high amounts, exacerbating the situation.

Gallstones

Copper is normally excreted from the body via the gallbladder. A reduction or blockage in gallbladder excretion can cause increased copper accumulation, even if copper intake is not excessive. Increased copper retention on the other hand can actually cause abnormal gallbladder function.

Estrogen is also known to affect gallbladder function, causing it to become sluggish. Estrogen is well known to contribute to cholesterol and calcium stone formation, and is probably the reason women are more prone to gallstone formation than men. It should also be noted that women have higher tissue copper levels than men.

Viral And Bacterial Infections

Viral infections produce a sedative response that slows down the metabolic rate. Bacterial infections, on the other hand, produce a stimulatory response, thereby increasing the metabolic rate. This is why people become feverish when they have a bacterial infection, but feel chilled when they have a virus. Low TMA copper levels are commonly seen in individuals with chronic bacterial infections, and elevated TMA copper levels typically accompany viral infections.

Excessive tissue copper levels are often seen in people who have had a severe viral condition such as hepatitis and mononucleosis. Following these infections, copper levels may remain elevated for years. The symptoms of fatigue, lethargy, and depression often linger as well.

High tissue copper predisposes an individual to recurring viral infections. This pattern is frequently seen in individuals who have been diagnosed with Epstein Barr, and/or cytomegleo virus. These viruses are known to be related to the Chronic Fatigue Syndrome (CFS). Often individuals with CFS will have great difficulty overcoming their condition unless they have their tissue copper levels evaluated and take appropriate measures to lower excessive levels.

The body's delicate balance of copper stores can predispose an individual to both viral, or bacterial infections. An example of how this works is to monitor the copper levels of menstruating women. As mentioned previously, copper is closely associated with the hormone estrogen. As a woman approaches her menstrual cycle, her estrogen level normally rises, as well as her copper level. This is why women are more susceptible to viral infections prior to menstruation. After menstruation, serum copper and estrogen levels normally fall, at which time they can become more susceptible to bacterial infections.

With this information, physicians can successfully treat

patients with these conditions. For example, any substance that antagonizes copper retention could be considered anti-viral. Substances that increase copper retention can help fight bacterial infections.

Nutrients such as zinc, vitamin A, and vitamin C have long been known for their ability to reduce viral infections. It is noteworthy that these nutrients are also known to antagonize copper.

Yeast And Fungus

People suffering from yeast and fungal conditions often have iron and zinc deficiencies. At the same time, their tissue copper levels are usually elevated above normal. Excessive concentrations of copper apparently produce an environment that encourages yeast and fungal proliferation. Individuals with chronic candidiasis typically have high tissue copper levels.

Therapy aimed at just controlling the spread of this condition may temporarily bring relief, but the condition soon returns unless a metabolic change is brought about. One of the most effective ways to eliminate the overgrowth of yeast and fungus is to reduce the high tissue copper accumulation. A well-balanced diet, along with the use of nutrients synergistic to zinc, but antagonistic to copper, helps to change the metabolic predisposition toward these conditions.

Scoliosis

Adequate amounts of copper are required for the normal production of elastin and collagen, which are the primary components of ligaments and the spinal discs. Copper specifically is necessary for the cross-linking of protein that gives strength and integrity to these structures. Zinc is required for the body to synthesize protein, therefore an imbalance between copper and zinc can lead to ligament and structural abnormalities.

High tissue copper is commonly found in patients with scoliosis. Scoliosis, a severe curvature of the spine, is a demoralizing condition that commonly strikes young girls, especially at puberty. Perhaps one of the reasons that this condition is so prevalent in young women is the copper-estrogen relationship. At puberty, estrogen levels normally rise along with an increase in tissue copper levels. If an individual already has a high copper level, the impending increase leads to a worsening of the scoliosis during this time. As estrogen and copper levels rise in tandem, the ligaments relax, thereby contributing to the advancement of the condition.

This same phenomenon occurs during pregnancy. Estrogen and copper levels soar during the course of pregnancy reaching their peak during the last trimester. This is normal and causes the pelvic ligaments to relax. The resulting elasticity makes it easier for the baby to travel through the birth canal.

Copper And Mental Function

Today nutritionists are studying how nutrition (or lack of it) affects brain function. Medical research is beginning to recognize that neurological function is very sensitive to one's nutritional status. Mental function is often the first thing to be affected by nutritional imbalances.

The brain stores trace elements in various sectors. An abnormal concentration or imbalance among these minerals can affect psychological functions, including emotions, memory, perception, learning and behavior.

Tissue zinc/copper ratios seem to affect brain hemisphere dominance. If the zinc portion of the ratio rises too high, the left brain, which controls verbal, analytical and sequential thinking, tries to take over. If the copper level surges past the zinc, the right hemisphere takes over, boosting creativity.

These variances show up clearly in the different genders. Men who are typically left brain types have more zinc than copper in their systems. An emotional woman who is extremely creative generally has elevated copper levels. Artists of both sexes usually have increased tissue copper levels, as do actors, and musicians. Intellectual types, on the other hand, often have elevated zinc levels.

Copper excess associated with hemisphere dominance is seen in children with dyslexia. Figure 20 shows the handwriting of an 11-year-old child who was diagnosed as having dyslexia and learning disability to the point that he had to be enrolled in special education classes. Unfortunately, this solution dealt with the result, but not the cause, of his problems. A TMA showed the typical low zinc-copper pattern. Fortunately, children with this condition respond well to nutritional supplements that correct this mineral imbalance. Figure 21 shows the dramatic change in this child's handwriting after three months on a specific, metabolic rebalancing nutritional program. The child enjoyed an improved attention span, better grades and more emotional stability. When school started the following September, he was able to be enrolled in regular classes. The student continued to perform well.

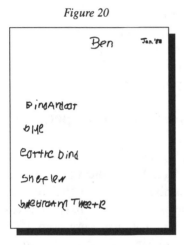

Figure 20

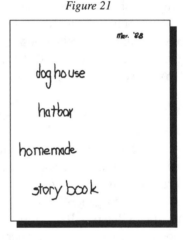

Figure 21

Dr. Richard Malter, a psychotherapist in Shaumberg, Ilinois, has dealt extensively with children having learning disabilities. Dr. Malter puts a great deal of emphasis on the biochemical basis of these and other behavioral disorders. He feels that this mineral relationship in children is having a tremendous impact upon our educational system. Dr. Malter explains, "In general, school curriculum tends to emphasize verbal analytical-sequential functions. If there is validity to the tissue Zn/Cu ratio and hemisphere dominance hypothesized by Dr. Watts, then any change in the dominance of the school population may have profound implications for our schools and the curriculum taught in them. If a shift in hemisphere dominance due to increasing copper accumulation from one generation to the next is developing, then our traditional left brain curriculum will become increasingly difficult for larger and larger numbers of children and adolescents.

This may be one of the reasons why there appears to be increasing numbers of learning disabled children in our schools' classrooms. Another way of looking at the problem is that our schools are becoming more and more out of synchronization with the children who are trying to learn. As this out-of-synch process continues, our schools are becoming more and more dysfunctional as systems of education. If this hypothesis is valid, two major implications should be considered. First, fundamental curriculum changes need to be made in the direction of right hemisphere functions. The other implication is to develop effective ways to educate the public and professionals to the problem of copper toxicity and how it may be reversed. If a child is having trouble in school due to learning disabilities, the first consideration should be to evaluate his/her nutritional status through a TMA." We have found mineral imbalances in countless children tested at our lab who were experiencing learning difficulties.

Medications That May Contribute To Copper Toxicity

The main excretion route for copper is through the intestinal track via the liver and gallbladder. Any medication that interferes with this excretion can contribute to copper toxicity. The hormone estrogen as well as some psychotropic drugs, sedatives, and tranquilizers will interrupt this elimination process. Some common drugs that can cause copper toxicity include thorazine, librium, norpramin, diuril, orinase, tegretol, tapazol and indocin.

Endocrine Effects Upon Copper

The body excretes excess copper via the liver when it receives the appropriate signals from the adrenal glands. When the sympathetic endocrines work overtime, they increase the body's metabolic rate. In turn, this increases copper elimination.

The para-sympathetic endocrine glands work in opposition to the sympathetic glands. The para-sympathetic endocrines thereby increase copper uptake and retention.

Copper And The Thyroid

Elevated tissue copper is a common finding with thyroid insufficiency or hypothyroidism. Copper has an antagonistic effect upon iron. If an iron deficiency develops, the thyroid will not function optimally.

Copper can also affect thyroid function through the actions of insulin. Elevated tissue copper increases the tissue retention of calcium, which triggers an increase in insulin secretion by the pancreas. Since zinc is required for the storage of insulin, it is possible that the zinc-copper antagonism could be responsible for flooding insulin into the blood.

Copper And The Adrenal Glands

Most individuals with weak adrenal glands will have high copper levels. This can be due to two factors. First, copper itself decreases adrenal gland activity similar to its effect upon the thyroid. Secondly, if the adrenals first become weak, then copper retention rises. Hormones from the adrenal glands normally stimulate the liver and thereby increase copper removal from the body. We often see poor liver function in individuals with high copper, resulting in chronic constipation. On the other hand, people with high adrenal and thyroid gland activity usually have normal to low tissue copper levels.

Factors Contributing To Copper Deficiency: Minerals

Figure 22 shows the minerals that are antagonistic to copper. Prolonged high intake of these elements, either taken together or in any combination, can produce a copper deficiency.

The nutritional minerals listed can also be used to treat copper toxicity. On the other hand, copper supplementation can help decrease the toxic effects of some heavy metals by inhibiting their absorption.

Figure 22
Minerals Antagonistic To Copper

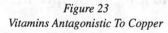

Vitamins

Vitamins antagonistic to copper are shown in figure 23. Any one can exacerbate an existing copper deficiency. The opposite can also occur. Excessive copper retention can produce a deficiency of any of these vitamins, thereby increasing their dietary requirements.

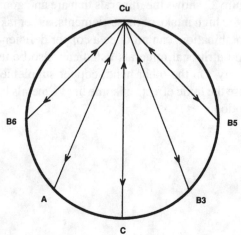

Figure 23
Vitamins Antagonistic To Copper

A lack of copper and a deficiency of Vitamin C have similar effects on the body. A copper deficiency mimics scurvy, causes bleeding gums, and bruising. Vitamin C requirements increase when an over abundance of copper builds up in the body. This increased demand for vitamin C can also lead to signs of scurvy.

Because vitamin C is antagonistic toward copper, it should NOT be taken in megadoses until a person's copper level has been evaluated. Vitamin C can be helpful to combat viral infections, which is why many Americans take their daily doses. But it should be noted that a copper deficient person can increase his/her susceptibility to bacterial infections by ingesting too much vitamin C.

Synergistic Nutrients

Synergistic vitamins include D, B_1, B_{12}, C and folic acid. Adding these synergistic vitamins to the diet can help restore the body's copper balance.

Calcium, cobalt, iron, selenium and sodium are minerals synergistic to copper. Copper aids in the retention of calcium and enhances vitamin D metabolism. When a copper deficiency or excess occurs, it sets off a chain reaction that can lead to an imbalance of other vitamins and minerals.

References

Mills, E.S: Idopathic Hypochromia. **Am. J. Med. Sci.,** 182, 1931.
Daniels, A.L., Wright, O.E: Iron and Copper Retention in Young Children. **J. Nutr.** 8, 1934.
Cartwright, G.E., Wintrobe, M.M: Copper Metabolism in Normal Subjects. **J. Clin. Nutr.** 14, 1964.
Klevay, L.M: Hair as a Biopsy Material. II Assessment of Copper Nutriture. **Am. J. Clin. Nutr.** 23, 1970.
Deeming, S.B., Weber, C.W: Hair Analysis of Trace Minerals in Human Subjects as Influenced by Age, Sex, and Oral Contraceptive Use. **Am. J. Clin. Nutr.** 31, 1978.
Vir, S.C., et al: Serum and Hair Concentrations of Copper During Pregnancy. **Am. J. Clin. Nutr.** 34, 1981.
IIkeda, T., et al: Hair Copper and Zinc Concentrations in Handicapped Children with Anticonvulsants. **Dev. Pharmacol. Ther.** 6, 1983.
Baumslag, N., et al: Trace Metal Content of Maternal and Neonate Hair. **Arch. Environ. Hlth.** 29, 1974.
Osaki, S., et al: The Mobilization of Iron from Perfused Mamalian Liver by Serum Copper Enzyme, Ferroxidase I. **J. Biol. Chem.** 246, 1971.
Fairbanks, V.F., et al: **Clinical Disorders of Iron Metabolism,** 2nd Ed. Grune & Straton, N.Y., 1971.
Mowat, A.G., Hothersall, T.E: Nature of Anaemia in Rheumatoid Arthritis. VII. Iron Content of Synovial Tissue in Patients with Rheumatoid Arthritis and in Normal Individuals. **Ann. Rheum. Dis.** 27, 1968.
Rainsford, K.D: Environmental Metal Ion Pertubations. Especially as They Affect Copper Status, are a Factor in the Etiology of Arthritic Conditions: An Hypothesis. **Inflammatory Disease and Copper.** Sorenson, J.R.J., Ed. Humana Press. N.J., 1982.
Mason, K.E: A Conspectus of Research on Copper Metabolism and Requirements of Man. **J. Nutr.** 109, 1979.
Chandra, R.H., Newberne, A.M: **Nutrition Immunity and Infections.** Plenum Press. N.Y., 1977.
Beisel, W.R: **The Effects of Infection on Host Nutritional Status.** Advances in Human Clinical Nutrition. Vitale, J.J., Broitman, S.A., Eds. John Wright, PSG., Inc. Boston, 1982.
Collie, W.R., et al: Hair in Menkes Disease: A Comprehensive Review. **Hair Trace Elements and Human Illness.** Brown, A.C., Crounse, R.G., Eds. Prager Pub. N.Y., 1980.

Dumont, A.E., et al: Siderosis of Lymph Nodes in Patients with Hodgkin's Disease. **Cancer** 38, 1976.

Sorenson, R.J., et al: Antineoplastic Activities of Some Copper Salicylates. **Trace Substances in Environmental Health XVI.** Hemphill, D.D., Ed. Univ. Mo., Columbia, 1982.

Dickerson, J.W.T: Nutrition of the Cancer Patient. **Advances in Nutritional Research** Vol. 5. Draper, H.H., Ed. Plenum Pub., N.Y., 1983.

Graham, G.C., Cordano, A: Copper Deficiency in Human Subjects. **Trace Elements in Human Health and Disease.** Prasad, A.S., Ed. Academic Press, N.Y., 1976.

Klevay, L.M: Coronary Heart Disease: The Zinc/Copper Hypothesis. **Am. J. Clin. Nutr.** 28, 1975.

Klevay, L.M: The Role of Copper and Zinc in Cholesterol Metabolism. **Advances in Nutritional Research.** Draper, H.H., Ed. Plenum Pub., N.Y., 1971.

Pratt, W.B., Phippen, W.G: Elevated Hair Copper Level in Idiopathic Scolosis, Preliminary Observations. **Spine** 5, 1980.

Douglas, et al: Trace Elements in Scalp-Hair of Persons with Multiple Sclerosis and of Normal Individuals. **Clin. Chem.** 24, 1978.

O'Dell, B.L: Biochemistry of Copper. **The Medical Clinics of North America.** 60, W.B. Saunders, Phil. 1960.

Finley, E.B., Cerklewski, Fl: Influences of Ascorbic Acid Supplementation on Copper Status in Young Adult Men. **Am. J. Clin. Nutr.** 37, 1983.

Schienberg, I.H., Sternlieb, I: Copper Toxicity and Wilson's Disease. **Trace Elements in Human Health and Disease.** Vol.I. Prasad, A.S., Ed. Academic Press. N.Y., 1976.

Watts, D.L: The Effects of Oral Contraceptive Agents on Nutritional Status. **Am. Chiro.** Mar., 1985.

Kirshnamachari, K: Some Aspects of Copper Metabolism in Pellagra. **Am. J. Clin. Nutr.** 27, 1967.

Bennion, L.J., et al: Effects of Oral Contraceptives on the Gallbladder Bile of Normal Women. **N.E.J.M.** 294, 1976.

Ingelfinger, F.J: Gallstones and Estrogens. **N.E.J.M.** 290, 1974.

Ockner, R.K., Davidson, C.S: Hepatic Effects of Oral Contraceptives. **N.E.J.M.** 285, 1971.

Chapter 8

Zinc

Scientists first discovered zinc was an essential nutrient for the growth of living organisms in 1869. The requirement for zinc in human health was proven in the early 1960's. It was discovered that zinc deficiency was a causative factor in delayed sexual development and stunted growth in men. Since then researchers have discovered that zinc is important in both male and female hormone production and plays a pivotal role in human health and disease. It has been found to be essential for the normal function of over 100 enzyme systems in the body.

The highest concentration of zinc is found in the eye and optic nerve. The skin also has a high concentration of zinc and can be a sensitive indicator of an individual's zinc status, since the body will often draw the mineral from peripheral tissues when needed elsewhere by the body. Zinc is also found in the adrenal glands, bone, brain, heart, kidneys, liver, muscles, prostate gland, spleen, and testes. A zinc deficiency can therefore adversely affect these organs that require zinc.

Zinc Deficiency

Signs of zinc deficiency vary from individual to individual. This may partially be due to the fact that zinc deficiency can be absolute or relative. An absolute deficiency is when the body has an increased requirement, along with a lack of intake, or increased loss of the mineral. Stress, illness, increased thyroid activity, hyperadrenal function, medications, or toxic metal accumulation can contribute to an absolute zinc deficiency.

A relative deficiency develops as a result of zinc loss from tissue storage sites. This may not necessarily be due to a lack of intake. A relative deficiency can be spotted on a TMA report when the zinc level is within the normal range, but is lower in ratio when compared to an antagonistic mineral such as copper or cadmium. A relative deficiency can be caused by underactivity of the adrenal, or thyroid glands, or an overactive parathyroid gland.

Skin Conditions

As mentioned previously, the skin can be one of the first areas to manifest a zinc deficiency. One of the most serious manifestations of a zinc deficiency is a genetic disorder called acrodermatitis enteropathica. This disease occurs in children and is the result of a serious zinc deficiency. The condition results in severe pustular, eczematous skin lesions and affects the mouth, face, groin, hands and feet. Zinc deficiency has also been found in individuals suffering from other diseases that involve the skin, such as lupus erythematosus, scleroderma, and psoriasis.

Stretch marks are a good indicator of zinc deficiency. Since the skin depends upon zinc for its normal integrity, a deficiency allows the skin to tear just below the surface, producing these stretch marks. These are actually scars that develop due to injury of the skin. Stretch marks are seen following mechanical stress on the skin. This is why it is common for them to develop after pregnancy, and in athletes such as body builders, who bulk up and put on weight. Both conditions put stress on the skin causing tightening. Stretch marks around the breasts are frequently seen in women who have zinc deficiency. The color of the stretch marks can give a clue as to an absolute or relative zinc deficiency. A relative deficiency produces white or silver stretch marks. Red or purple lines are a sign of an absolute zinc deficiency.

Generally speaking, zinc deficiency can contribute to skin blemishes and rashes, as well as slower healing of wounds.

Nails

The fingernails can also indicate one's zinc status. White spots on the nails can be a sign of zinc deficiency. These spots may develop after a viral infection or following a fast. Actually, these spots are more often caused by too much copper, which is a potent antagonist to zinc.

Sickle Cell Anemia

It has been discovered that individuals suffering from sickle cell anemia have a marked zinc deficiency. In the course of this disease, excessive calcium accumulates within the red blood cells. This causes the cell to become rigid and misshapened or deformed. Zinc is beneficial for this condition and helps to decrease the infiltration of calcium into the red cells. TMA studies have shown low zinc levels relative to copper in patients who suffer from sickle cell anemia or who have the sickle cell trait.

Diabetes

Insulin storage requires adequate amounts of available zinc. Zinc depletion is found generally in all forms of diabetes, but most notably in the juvenile type.

Anorexia Nervosa

It is possible that zinc deficiency may play a role in the development of this devastating eating disorder. Anorexia nervosa is more common among women than men. It is thought to be psychogenic in origin, being especially prevalent among women in their teens. However, two components of anorexia are taste disorders and loss of smell, classic signs of zinc deficiency. The development of zinc deficiency may be related to excessive copper accumulation.

As young girls begin to mature and enter puberty, their copper levels normally rise along with the female hormone estrogen. As their copper levels rise, so does their need for zinc. If they do not obtain sufficient amounts of zinc from their diets, a deficiency will result. A number of factors can contribute to an increase of copper burden, such as the use of oral contraceptive agents, estrogen therapy, a lack of protein intake, illness, and stress. All of these factors are common ingredients in the lifestyles of female college students, which may explain the high incidence of anorexia among this group.

Menstrual Irregularities

It is very common to find zinc-copper imbalances in patients with menstrual irregularities. Copper is related to the female hormone estrogen and zinc is related to progesterone. TMA studies of female patients complaining of pre- and post menstrual irregularities show a disturbance in their zinc/copper ratios. This indicates a disturbance in their estrogen/progesterone ratio as well. A low zinc/copper ratio is related to a progesterone deficit relative to estrogen. This TMA pattern is typical in patients with premenstrual syndrome. Their periods are usually heavy and may be prolonged, with accompanying symptoms of fatigue, depression, weight gain, frontal headaches, constipation, and food cravings. A high TMA zinc/copper ratio indicates an estrogen deficit relative to progesterone, as zinc aids in progesterone production. Women with this pattern often feel better premenstrually and yet can experience symptoms immediately following menstruation. We call this the post-menstrual syndrome. Symptoms can include anxiety, defensiveness, indecision, agitated depression, fluid retention and breast soreness.

Viruses

A lack of zinc is associated with a decrease in immune response and increased susceptibility to infections. Viruses are known to contribute to zinc deficiency. This trace element however also possesses anti-viral properties. Zinc can destroy some viruses on contact. Vitamin A, the anti-infectious vitamin, in combination with zinc, can be a powerful foe against many types of viruses.

The list on the following page summarizes other conditions that have been associated with zinc deficiency either absolute or relative based upon TMA studies.

RELATIVE ZINC DEFICIENCY	ABSOLUTE ZINC DEFICIENCY
AIDS	Macular Degeneration
Autism	Manic Depression
Candida	Peptic Ulcers
Depression	Prostate Enlargement
Eclampsia	Rheumatoid Arthritis
Fungus	Sterility
Gastric Ulcers	Immune Suppression
Premenstrual Syndrome	Loss of Smell and Taste
Post Partum Depression	Slow Wound Healing
Pregnancy	
Viruses	
Immune Deficiency	

Why A Zinc Deficiency Develops

Medications can contribute to a deficiency of zinc by suppressing its absorption, increasing its excretion or by interfering with synergistic nutrients, such as magnesium and vitamin B_6. Some of the more common drugs that adversely affect zinc status are anti-depressants, anti-inflammatory medications such as cortisone and prednisone, as well as diuretics.

Foods containing high amounts of phytic acid bind with the zinc molecules, making it difficult, if not impossible, for the body to absorb the mineral. Grains in general and unleavened breads in particular, are high in phytates. Many vegetarians have increased zinc requirements because of their high fiber diets.

Alcoholics also frequently develop zinc deficiency. Alcohol causes the body to lose critical stores through the kidneys.

Zinc Overload

Excessive intake of zinc over prolonged periods can produce dangerous deficiencies in other minerals. The most dangerous toxicity problem is an elevated zinc level relative to copper. If this ratio is skewed, high cholesterol levels can develop, contributing to cardiovascular disease. When zinc is excessively high relative to copper, the low density lipoproteins (LDL) are increased, and the high density lipoproteins (HDL) become markedly reduced. Adequate HDL levels help in preventing fat deposition within the arteries and should always be higher than the LDLs.

Zinc is necessary for a normal immune response, although too much zinc relative to copper can also compromise the immune system. As mentioned in a previous chapter, copper deficiency increases the tendency toward bacterial infections.

Minerals And Vitamins Antagonistic To Zinc

Many nutritional factors affect zinc status. Figure 24 shows the minerals that are antagonistic to zinc. Excessive intake or increased tissue retention of any one or combination of these can contribute to a zinc deficiency. They can prevent the body from using zinc properly or interfere with its absorption.

Excessive accumulation or toxicity of any of the elements in figure 24 can be treated with zinc therapy since the antagonism is mutual. This is why zinc has been especially useful in combatting the adverse effects of toxic heavy metals like cadmium, mercury, and lead.

Figure 24
Minerals Antagonistic To Zinc

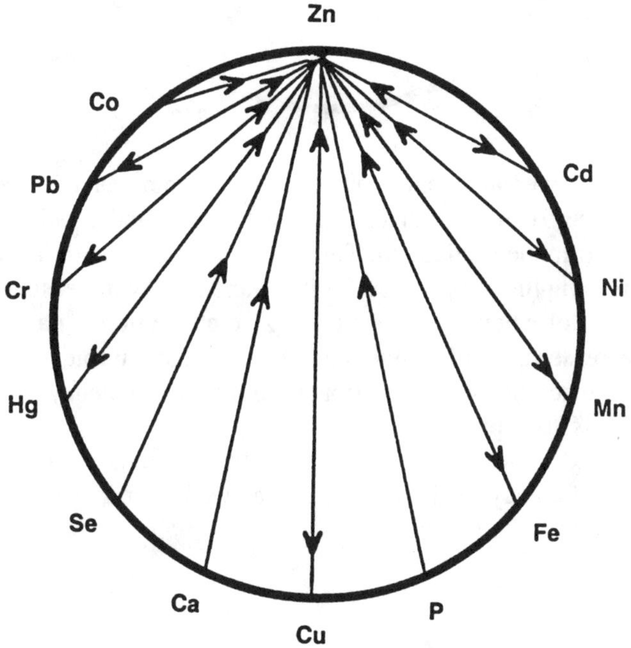

Vitamins can affect zinc status as well. Vitamins considered antagonistic to zinc are listed in figure 25.

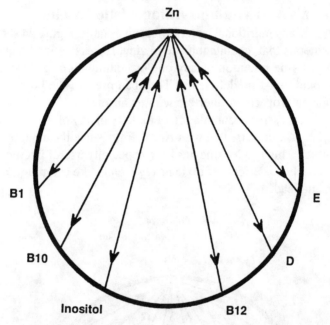

Figure 25
Vitamins Antagonistic To Zinc

An over abundant intake of these vitamins can affect zinc in a number of ways. For example, vitamin E and B_1 stimulate adrenal hormone production. This can produce a zinc deficiency by increasing the body's need for it. Vitamin D, by increasing the absorption of calcium, can suppress zinc absorption. Vitamin D also decreases thyroid activity and increases parathyroid activity. This sequence of events contributes to a zinc deficiency by decreasing its absorption.

Excessive zinc intake, on the other hand, can produce a relative deficiency of these minerals, as well as increase the requirement of these vitamins.

Synergistic Nutrients

Magnesium, iron, and phosphorus work in concert with zinc. So do vitamins A, B_1, B_3, B_5, B_6, and E.

There is a fine line between synergism and antagonism. Depending upon the individual, a certain amount of a mineral or vitamin can help the body metabolize zinc. But, if the concentration gets too high, it can hinder or halt the absorption, or interfere with zinc activated enzymes. Copper for example, is antagonistic to zinc. The two, however, must be present in a proper relationship in order to work together to build and maintain connective tissue.

Tissue Mineral Analysis (TMA) And Zinc Analysis

TMA of the hair is considered one of the best methods for determining long term nutritional zinc status. However, the hair is not a sensitive indicator of acute zinc depletion. Traditional tests such as plasma, serum, and red blood cell levels are also not good indicators of zinc status because zinc is an intracellular element. As with most minerals, the body maintains the blood levels at the expense of the tissues. The blood then is the last to reflect a chronic mineral deficiency.

It is also difficult to determine if the zinc level found in the serum or plasma represents zinc status or tissue redistribution. The body routinely takes zinc from one tissue site, such as the skin, and redistributes it to another organ that has a greater requirement. This is why a person may show a normal or even high blood zinc level and still be suffering from a zinc deficiency. Other than through TMA, the only way to unconditionally determine a zinc deficiency is through response to zinc therapy.

Zinc Requirements

The established minimum daily requirements for zinc are three to five milligrams per day for infants. Grown women need about 20 milligrams daily unless they are lactating. At that time the requirements jump to twenty-five milligrams. Men need at least 15 milligrams.

However, many other factors can affect these requirements. Stress levels, for example, can raise the need for more zinc. Medications, infections, or an exclusive vegetarian diet can increase zinc requirements as well.

Caution should be used when taking zinc supplements, especially if a person has an absolute requirement. They usually require only a small amount compared to those with a relative deficiency. People suffering relative deficiencies frequently have astronomical zinc requirements that can be several times the minimum daily requirement. A person tends to respond best to zinc therapy when other antagonistic and synergistic nutrients are used appropriately.

We have seen individuals develop serious problems when they take zinc supplements indiscriminately. I recall a physician who was worried about his enlarged prostate. He read an article mentioning that zinc deficiency can contribute to this condition, which is true. So he began taking 150 milligrams of zinc each day. His prostate condition did indeed improve. As a precautionary measure, he continued taking this amount daily for over a year. He later developed an enlargement of his prostate, and naturally since 150 milligrams of zinc was not helping the condition, he doubled his supplement intake to 300 milligrams daily. However, his condition got much worse instead of better. How could this happen? What happened was this: His prolonged zinc intake created a copper deficiency. When the body is short of copper, it is primed for a potential bacterial infection. This time his prostate problem was caused by an infection and was not simply a prostate enlargement. The zinc supplements he had been taking for over a year may have actually contributed to, and even intensified, the prostate infection. Even when he began taking antibiotics along with the zinc, there was a steady worsening of his condition. After speaking with him and learning about his history of taking zinc supplements, my first thought was that he had induced a copper deficiency. I suggested that he suspend the zinc supplements immediately, and send a hair sample for analysis. In the meantime I advised him to begin taking a copper supplement, approximately 8 milligrams per day. Within three days his prostatitis markedly improved. His hair analysis test confirmed the copper deficiency.

This is not an unusual story. People think of nutritional supplements like money: If some is good, more is even better. Not so. Balance is the more critical factor in body chemistry.

References

Prasad, A.S., et al: Biochemical Studies on Dwarfism, Hypogonadism and Anemia. **AMA Arch. Intern. Med.** 111, 1963.

Prasad, A.S., et al: Zinc Metabolism in Patients with the Syndrome of Iron Deficiency Anemia, Hypogonadism, and Dwarfism. **J. Lab. Clin. Med.** 61, 1963.

Prasad, A.S: Metabolism of Zinc and its Deficiency in Human Subjects. **Zinc Metabolism.** Prasad, Ed. Charles Thomas Pub., Ill. 1966.

Hambridge, K.M., Walravens, P.A: Zinc Deficiency in Infants and Preadolescent Children. **Trace Elements in Human Health and Disease.** Prasad, Ed. Academic Press, N.Y. 1976.

Sandstead, H.H., Vo-Khactu, K.P., Solomons, N: Conditioned Zinc Deficiencies. **Trace Elements in Human Health and Disease.** Prasad, Ed. Academic Press. N.Y. 1976.

Hess, F.M., King, J.C., Margen, S: Zinc Excretion in Young Women on Low Zinc Intakes and Oral Contraceptive Agents. **J. Nutr.** 107, 1977.

Sanstead, H.H., et al: Zinc Nutriture: Effects on Lipid Metabolism and Plasma Zinc. **Clin. Res.** 28, 1980.

Sanstead, H.H: Zinc in Human Nutrition. **Disorders of Mineral Metabolism,** Vol. I. Bronner, F., Coburn, J., Eds. Academic Press, N.Y., 1981.

Hambidge, K.M., et al: Zinc Nutritional Status During Pregnancy: A longtitudinal Study. **Am. J. Clin. Nutr.** 37, 1983.

Neldner, K.H., Hambidge, K.M: Zinc Therapy of Acrodermatitis Enteropathica. **N.E.J.M.** 1975.

Prasad, A.S., et al: Zinc Deficiency in Sickle Cell Disease. **Clin. Chem.** 21, 1975.

Leopold, I.H: Zinc Deficiency and Visual Disturbance. **Am. J. Opthamal.** 85, 1978.

Pfeiffer, C.C: **Mental and Elemental Nutrients.** Keats Pub. Conn. 1975.

Netter, F.H., Forsham, P.H: **Endocrine System and Selected Metabolic Diseases.** Ciba Pharm., Col. Colorpress, N.Y. 1965.

Becker, W.M., Hoekstra, W.G: The Intestinal Absorption of Dietary Zinc. Intestinal Absorption of Metal Ions. **Trace Elements and Radionuclides.** Waldron, Edwards, Eds. Pergamon Press, Oxford, 1971.

Sandstead, H.H: Interactions of Cadmium and Lead With Essential Minerals. **Effects and Dose Response Relationships of Toxic Metals.** Nordberg, F.F., Ed. Elsevier, Amsterdam. 1976.

Davies, J.T: **The Clinical Significance of the Essential Biological Metals.** C. Thomas Pub. Springfield, Ill. 1972.

Chapter 9

Iron

Biochemical imbalances can create eating disorders — even bizarre behavior. One of the strangest eating disorders is pica.

One patient developed a habit of chewing pieces of paper. This happened gradually, without any real reason that she could pinpoint. Eventually, her appetite for paper grew. Her desire to chew paper turned into an uncontrollable desire to actually eat paper. She would snack on pages from paperback novels when the passages got steamy. If the heroine died and she began to cry, she would eat the tissue paper, and even the box when the tissues ran out. When she went to the movies she would not only eat the candy, but the wrappers as well.

This woman suffered from paper pica. Pica is a term that denotes an abnormal craving for substances other than food. The condition creates an irresistible desire to ingest paper as well as other non-food items. The cause: iron deficiency. This lady suffered from iron deficiency anemia, and as a result of eating paper, developed a mercury toxicity, since mercury is used to preserve paper products.

These two trace element conditions created a fertile atmosphere for paper pica to prosper. However, the cure was simple. Oral iron therapy completely eliminated her cravings for paper.

In the 1950's, Lawrence Welk made iron deficiency, or iron poor blood, a household word. Even today, the World Health

Organization labels iron deficiency as the world's major nutritional problem.

Anemia is a lack of the oxygen carrying red blood cells. Iron deficiency, however, can cause a host of other health problems since it is involved in many metabolic processes. In fact, iron deficiency without anemia is more prevalent than iron deficiency with anemia. Anemia accounts for only one-third of the problems caused by iron deficiency.

Mental Effects Of Iron

Scientific studies have discovered a correlation between iron status and intellectual performance. A lack of iron can lead to a shortened attention span, a reduction in cognitive functions, minimal brain dysfunction, and hyperactivity.

Disturbances in mental function can be caused by flaws in the metabolic pathways that require iron. Some of these defects are simply due to the effects of too little oxygen reaching the brain. Other disturbances can be due to DNA abnormalities, since the synthesis of DNA requires iron. A deficiency of iron can impair neuronal development. Iron is also necessary for the activation of enzymes involved in brain neurotransmitters.

Thousands of TMA studies have revealed that individuals with increased tissue iron levels are intellectually oriented. They are more apt to carry slide rules than football helmets. Their intellectual aptitude indicates left brain dominance. Not surprisingly, EEG studies of iron deficient patients confirm increased left hemisphere activity. It has also been observed that too much tissue iron accumulation may lead to aggressive behavior, as well as hostility and hyperactivity.

Other Conditions Associated With Iron Imbalance

One of the earliest recorded therapeutic uses of iron dates back to 500 B.C. The ancients used iron to treat a condition they called "chlorosis," which was diagnosed in individuals having pallor of the skin, swelling, palpitations of the heart, rapid pulse, prolonged sleep, cessation of the menses, and an aversion to eating. The condition was also described as creating a "heavy" feeling to the body and especially in the arms and legs.

The ancients were accurate. Twentieth century physicians have added other symptoms to this condition. These include intracranial hypertension, which can result in chronic dull headaches. Enlargement of organs such as the spleen and heart may also develop, as well as spoon shaped distortion of the fingernails. When anemia is present, the sclera of the eye may become pearly white or blue, and the nails may become brittle with ridges running lengthwise.

Pica

As discussed previously, pica is a term used to describe an abnormal or unusual craving for substances other than food. These cravings may include not only paper, but dirt, clay, rubber, and even laundry starch. The condition affects mostly women and children and is associated with iron deficiency. Pica is more common in poor rural areas or underdeveloped countries of the world. But, it is not strictly a socioeconomic problem and can strike anyone who has an iron problem.

The most common form of pica is geophagia, which is the ingestion of clay or dirt. This form is frequently seen in young children.

Pagophagia is the compulsive desire to chew ice. This fetish is usually seen in adults.

Amylophagia is a craving for starch, such as laundry starch. This condition often plagues pregnant and nursing women.

These different forms of pica are all indications of an iron imbalance and almost always respond to iron therapy.

Dysphagia

Dysphagia is a term that means difficulty in swallowing. If a person has difficulty swallowing pills for instance, it would be a good idea to have his or her iron status checked. Dysphagia is due to tightening of the esophagus and usually responds to iron therapy. If the thyroid gland is underactive, it can develop a goiter. This can put mechanical pressure on the esophagus restricting the ability to swallow. As will be discussed later, there is a close relationship between the thyroid gland and iron status. A frequent need to clear the throat, particularly when under stress, is a classic sign of possible low thyroid activity and low iron status.

Iron deficiency is known to weaken the immune system, making the body more susceptible to infections. This is probably due to accompanying nutritional deficiencies. Many diverse factors can contribute to iron deficiency. Pregnant mothers have an increased need for iron. Excessive blood loss can create a deficiency. Women are more susceptible to iron deficiency due to the losses that occur during monthly menstruation. Low iron intake, poor absorption, parasites, improper nutrition, medications, and other vitamin and mineral deficiencies can all contribute to an imbalance in one's iron status.

Iron And Infections

During a bacterial infection, the body shifts iron from the blood into storage compartments such as bone, liver, spleen, and lymphatic tissues. This is a protective measure that makes the iron unavailable to the bacteria, which needs iron for its growth.

This action, however, prevents the body from incorporating iron into the red blood cells. If the infection becomes chronic, it can create a type of anemia called "infectious anemia." This type of anemia is not due to an iron deficiency per se, but is due to the iron being locked in storage tissues. This type of anemia will not respond to iron therapy until the infection is brought under control, then the iron can be reutilized once more. Chronic infectious anemia can be spotted as an elevated iron to copper ratio on a TMA study. Many times the infection can be present for years. The most common type of infection of this nature is dental abscess.

Sequestering of iron into storage tissue also occurs in other conditions, such as rheumatoid arthritis, diabetes, and some types of malignancies. These conditions are known to cause anemia, even though the tissue concentrations of iron are more than adequate. It has been found that in patients with rheumatoid arthritis, iron can accumulate not only in soft tissues, but within the joints as well. The pancreas can accumulate iron to the point that normal insulin activity becomes impaired, and diabetes ensues. People frequently develop this condition following a serious bacterial infection.

Iron Overload

Iron overload affects men more often than women. There are two types of iron overload, called hemosiderosis and hemochromatosis. Hemosiderosis is described as a general increase in tissue iron without tissue destruction. Hemochromatosis is more serious, as iron accumulation results in damage to the liver, spleen, and pancreas. Iron deposits have also been found in the heart, joints, lymph nodes, skin, and even in the brain.

Iron overload can be caused by the ingestion of too much iron over long periods. Acute iron toxicity is the second most common cause of accidental poisoning in small children. The cause is usually due to consuming large quantities of iron supplements. Liver disease such as cirrhosis, hemolytic conditions, which is an abnormal destruction of red blood cells, and even multiple blood transfusions can lead to iron overload.

Probably the most well-known incidence of iron overload has been reported in the Bantu tribes of Africa, who brew and consume large quantities of homemade beer. Iron pots are used for the brewing, and the acidity of the beer has been found to leach large amounts of iron from the pots. Researchers found that the Bantu daily iron intake was over 200 milligrams. It has also been found that cooking in iron skillets or pots can increase the iron content of foods by as much as 400 percent. This would be perfectly all right for those who need extra iron, but for those who have a problem with increased iron accumulation, cooking in iron utensils should be avoided.

Water can also be a source of iron in regions with high iron soils. Older homes with iron plumbing can add to one's iron intake. If the porcelain in your sinks or toilet becomes stained a dark brown, chances are you have a high iron content in your water.

This was the source of a problem for a doctor and his wife. After retirement they moved to a farm and the house was quite old. Their water came from a well. In order to improve the taste of their water, they installed a filter on their faucets. After living there for a couple of years, they began experiencing many health problems. Their symptoms included migraine headaches, high blood pressure, and joint pain, to mention a few. Their TMAs revealed that they both had high tissue iron levels. The question was then asked, where did this iron come from? A water analysis was suggested. Two water samples were taken. One water sample was taken before it was filtered, and the other after it was run through the filter. The unfiltered water was of course high in iron, but surprisingly, the iron content was much higher in the filtered sample. Apparently they had not changed the charcoal filter since it was installed. The filter had built up a great deal of iron. When the filter became cracked from old age, it began dumping large amounts of iron into their drinking water.

Herbs can contribute significantly to iron intake. Peppermint, chickweed, comfrey root, licorice root and golden seal have high iron levels. These herbs can be helpful for those who need extra iron.

Alcohol is known to increase iron absorption. Excess iron is known to contribute to cirrhosis of the liver, which is common with alcoholism. Certain beverages are high iron as well, for example, red wines and imported dark beers. This may be why many people get headaches when they drink dark wines, but do not suffer if they drink white wine, which is low in iron.

Researchers have found that an imbalance of iron to copper may play a role in Parkinson's disease as well as other neurological disorders. People who died of Parkinson's disease were found to have increased iron accumulation and low copper levels in areas of the brain that is affected in this condition. This excess iron has also been found in patients with ALS (amyotrophic lateral sclerosis) also known as Lou Gehrig's disease. Tissue damage caused by excess iron is due to its effect of generating free radicals or lipid peroxidation. Copper, on the other hand, protects from this type of free radical formation in neurological tissues.

Iron and copper are closely related. Iron cannot be utilized by the body without adequate copper reserves. A person with a copper deficiency will retain iron because the body will stop eliminating it. If this person also ingests large amounts of vitamin C, the iron overload will multiply further as vitamin C enhances iron absorption, while antagonizing copper absorption.

The Endocrine (Hormonal) Effects Of Iron Imbalance

In 1938 physicians discovered a relationship between iron deficiency and hypothyroidism. Cecil stated that both thyroid therapy along with iron therapy was indicated for the treatment of anemia. Today researchers have found that iron deficiency can in fact impair thyroid function. The amino acid L-phenylalanine is normally converted to L-tyrosine which is the precursor to the thyroid hormone thyroxine. It has been found that this conversion is reduced by 50 percent in iron deficient patients. For this reason, low iron stores can be a good indicator for the potential development of low thyroid activity.

Since there is a reciprocal relationship between the thyroid and adrenal glands, it is possible that iron status may also reflect adrenal activity. Tissue mineral studies have shown that increased activity of the para-thyroid glands can contribute to iron deficiency. This can occur because the para-thyroid hormone increases the absorption of calcium, which is antagonistic to iron absorption.

A lack of pancreatic enzyme production can cause an increase in iron absorption. Pancreatic enzymes are often helpful in lowering excessive tissue iron build-up.

Minerals Antagonistic To Iron

Figure 26 lists the minerals that are considered antagonistic to iron. Excessive intake of any one or a combination of these trace elements can contribute to iron deficiency and ultimately anemia. They may also exacerbate an existing deficiency.

Deficiency of iron's synergistic trace elements can also lead to iron deficiency. The synergistic minerals include:

Copper (Cu)	Chromium (Cr)
Sodium (Na)	Nickel (Ni)
Selenium (Se)	Potassium (K)
Manganese (Mn)	Phosphorus (P)

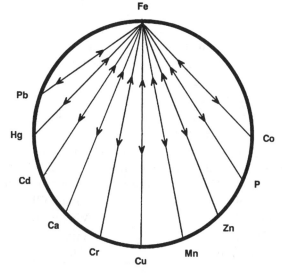

Figure 26
Minerals Antagonistic To Iron

Vitamins Antagonistic To Iron

Vitamins considered antagonistic to iron are listed in figure 27.

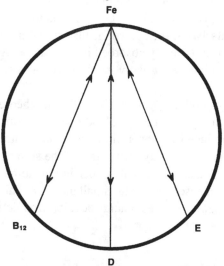

Figure 27
Vitamins Antagonistic To Iron

The antagonism of iron by these vitamins can be direct or a byproduct of another process. For example, vitamin D enhances the absorption of calcium, which inhibits iron absorption. Cobalt, an integral part of vitamin B_{12}, competes with iron absorption.

The antagonistic effects of iron and vitamin E occur on a cellular level. Vitamin E increases the metabolic demands for iron, while excess tissue iron increases the body's anti-oxidant requirements for vitamin E.

When a person develops an iron deficiency, s/he typically has a lack of other synergistic vitamins. A single mineral deficienciey rarely develops. Conversely, a shortage of synergistic vitamins can cause an iron deficiency and may be required to correct the iron imbalance. Synergistic vitamins to iron include:

Vitamin E	Vitamin B_6
Vitamin B_1	Vitamin B_{12}
Vitamin B_2	Vitamin C
Vitamin B_3	Vitamin A

Iron Requirements

Body tissues contain approximately 25 milligrams per kilogram or 2.2 pounds in adult women and 35 milligrams per kilogram in adult men. Iron's recommended daily intake (RDA) is 10 to 15 milligrams for infants and children, 10 milligrams for adult males, 18 milligrams for teenagers and adult women, and 45 milligrams for women who are pregnant or nursing.

The most absorbable type of iron is found in animal proteins, particularly red meats. Iron is also found in vegetables and grains, but it is not readily absorbed if eaten alone. Adding animal protein to the plate will greatly increase iron absorption from the diet.

Dairy products, especially milk and cheese, can reduce iron absorption by as much as 60 percent. Tea consumption will also readily reduce iron absorption due to its tannic acid content.

The body can only utilize iron if the stomach has an acid environment. A lack of normal acidity in the stomach will markedly reduce iron absorption in the small intestine. This is why many people who regularly take antacids develop iron deficiency.

References

Vitale, J.J: Impact of Nutrition on Immune Function. **Advances in Human Clinical Nutrition.** Vitale, Broitman, Eds. John Wright, Inc. Boston, 1982.
Alpers, D.H, Clouse, R.E., Stenson, W.F: **Manual of Nutritional Therapeutics.** Little Brown and Co. Boston, 1983.
Fielding, J., et al: Iron Deficiency Without Anemia. **Lancet** 2, 1965.
Heinrich, H.C: Iron Deficiency Without Anemia. **Lancet,** 1968.
Prasad, A.S: **Trace Elements and Iron in Human Metabolism.** Plenum Pub. N.Y., 1978.
Webb, T.E., Oski, F.A: Iron Deficiency Anemia and Scholastic Achievement in young adolescents. **J. Ped.** 82, 1973.
Oskie, F.A., Honig, A.M: The Effects of Therapy on the Development Scores of Iron-Deficient Infants. **J. Ped.,** 92, 1978.
Tucker, D.M., et al: Iron Status and Brain Function: Serum Ferritin Levels Associated with Asymmetries of Cortical Electro-physiology and Cognitive Performance. **Am. J. Clin. Nutr.** 39, 1984.
Pollitt, E., et al: Iron Deficiency and Behavorial Development in Infants and Preschool Children. **Am. J. Clin. Nutr.** 43, 1986.
Cantwell, R.J: The Long Term Neurological Sequelae of Anemia in Infancy. **Ped. Res.** 8, 1974.
Voorhess, M.L., et al: Iron Deficiency Anemia and Increased Urinary Norepinephrine Excretion. **J. Ped.** 86, 1975.
Tucker, D.M., et al: Neuropsychological Effects of Iron Deficiency. **Neurobiology of the Trace Elements,** Vol.I. Dreosti, Smith, Eds. Humana Press N.Y., 1983.
Lindenbaum, J: The Hematopoietic System. **Nutrition, Metabolic and Clinical Applications.** Hodges, R.E., Ed. Plenum Press. N.Y., 1979.
Gutelius, M.F., et al: Nutritional Studies of Children with Pica II. Treatment of Pica with Iron given Intramuscularly. **Ped.** 29, 1962.
Reynolds, R.D., et al: Pagophagia and Iron Deficiency Anemia. **Ann. Intern. Med.** 69, 1968.
Roselle, H.A: Association of Laundry Starch and Clay Ingestion with Anemia in New York City. **Arch. Int. Med.** 125, 1970.
Dillman, E., et al: Hypothermia in Iron Deficiency due to Altered Triiodothyronine Metabolism. **Am. J. Physiol.** 239, 1980.
Lehmann, W.D., Henrich, H.C: Impaired Phenylalanine-Tyrosine Conversion in Patients with Iron-Deficiency Anemia Studied by a L-(2H5)Phenylalanine-Loading Test. **Am. J. Clin. Nutr.** 44, 1986.

Fairbanks, V.F., et al: **Clinical Disorders of Iron Metabolism,** 2nd. Ed. Grune and Stratton. N.Y., 1971.

Brown, J.: **Integration and Coordination of Metabolic Processes. A Systems Approach to Endocrinology.** Van Norstrand Reinhold Co. N.Y., 1978.

Beisel, W.R., et al: The Impact of Infectious Disease on Trace Element Metabolism on the Host. **Trace Element Metabolism in Animals,** Vol 2. Hoekstra, Suttie, Ganther, Eds. Univ.Park Press. Baltimore, 1974.

MacDougall, L.G., et al: The Immune Response in Iron Deficient Children: Impaired Cellular Defense Mechanisms with Altered Humoral Components. **J. Ped.** 86, 1975.

Chandra, R.K., Newbern, P.M: **Nutrition, Immunity, and Infection. Mechanisms of Interactions.** Plenum Press. N.Y., 1977.

Flanagan, P.R., et al: Increased Dietary Cadmium Absorption in Mice and Human Subjects with Iron Deficiency. **Gastroenterol.** 74, 1978.

Pollack, S., et al: The Absorption of Nonferrous Metals in Iron Deficiency. **J. Clin. Invest.** 44, 1965.

Kirchgessner, M., et al: **Interactions of Essential Metals in Human Physiology. Clinical, Biochemical, and Nutritional Aspects of Trace Elements.** Alan R. Liss, Inc. N.Y., 1982.

Aust, S.D, White, B.C: Iron Chelation Prevents Tissue Injury Following Ischemia. **Advances in Free Radical Biology and Medicine** Vol.I. Pryor, W.A., Ed. Pergamin Press. N.Y., 1985.

Williams, M.L., et al: Role of Dietary Iron and Fat on Vitamin E Deficiency Anemia of infancy. **N.E.J.M.** 292, 1975.

Saunders, S.J., et al: Iron Absorption in Pancreatic Disease. **Lancet** ii, 1962.

Dexter, D.T., et al: Increased Nigral Iron Content in Postmortem Parkinsonian Brains. **Lancet,** ii 1987.

Dexter, D., et al: Lipid Peroxidation as a Cause of Nigral Cell Death in Parkinsons Disease. **Lancet,** 1986.

Chapter 10

Manganese

A well-known professional basketball player was a devout vegetarian. He felt he performed better if he kept to a strict vegetarian diet. However, while his shooting and concentration seemed improved, he kept breaking bones, which then healed very, very, slowly. His joints also became increasingly unstable. His basketball career seemed to be at a halt.

Eventually, his physicians discovered he had no detectable manganese in his system. They immediately prescribed manganese supplements. Over a period of several months his bones began to mend, making him strong enough to return to the NBA court.

Manganese is distributed throughout most of the body's tissues. The highest concentrations are found in the bone, kidneys, liver, pituitary, pancreas and thyroid.

Lowered levels have been found in patients suffering from Down's syndrome, epilepsy and schizophrenia. Elevated levels have been found in patients with multiple sclerosis, learning disabilities and Parkinson's disease.

In contemporary America, manganese deficiency appears to be as prevalent as iron deficiency. After years of TMA testing, we routinely have found low manganese levels in the hair of patients with hypoglycemia (low blood sugar), hypothyroidism, adrenal insufficiency, kidney problems, and diabetes.

How Your Body Utilizes Manganese

Manganese is located largely in the mitochondria. The mitochondria are tiny compartments within our cells that produce most of the body's energy. They are often referred to as the power houses of the cell. The structure and function of these mitochondria are particularly affected by our manganese status. A disturbance in manganese status can produce adverse energy production, leading to overall fatigue.

Manganese is a constituent in some enzymes and activates others. This trace element activates enzymes associated with fatty acid metabolism, carbohydrate metabolism, and protein synthesis. Manganese plays a very important roll in protecting cells from damage due to free radical production, particularly superoxide radicals. Manganese activates the free radical scavenger, superoxide dismutase, within the cellular mitochondria.

Hormonal Effects Upon Manganese

Normal thyroid function requires manganese, since it is involved with the formation of thyroxin, the thyroid's most important hormone. Tissue mineral analysis studies have revealed low manganese levels in patients with an inactive thyroid. Absorption or utilization of manganese may be impaired when the body's estrogen, insulin or parathyroid hormone levels are elevated, since they are antagonistic to thyroid function.

The adrenal hormones affect the tissue distribution of manganese and they can also alter its metabolism.

Manganese And Diet

Tissue manganese levels are directly related to the substance's availability in the diet. Even though vegetables are generally high in manganese, a vegetarian diet does not necessarily improve manganese levels. Foods having a high phytic acid content can inhibit manganese absorption.

Meat, on the other hand, is not a high source of manganese. However, scientific studies have found that subjects eating a high protein diet have a healthier manganese status than those eating a diet low in protein. Meat enhances the bio-availability of manganese in the diet. Therefore, eating meat with vegetables high in manganese assures that the body will be able to absorb enough manganese.

Although tea is rich in manganese, it is unavailable for absorption because of the tannin content of the drink. Alcohol, on the other hand, increases the liver's manganese level and apparently doubles its absorption.

Manganese Deficiency

Skeletal abnormalities, postural defects and impaired growth are common in patients who have a shortage of manganese. Retarded bone growth, which causes bowing, can occur. Tendon problems, osteoporosis or "brittle bones" are other common conditions. Sufferers of adult Down's syndrome frequently develop secondary hip joint dislocations; doctors suspect this condition to be related to manganese deficiency.

Manganese deficiency can indirectly lead to cartilage and connective tissue disorders. Therefore, conditions such as Osgood Schlaters, Perthes disease, and lupus may benefit from manganese.

Impaired reproductive functions can also result from a manganese deficiency. Defective ovulation, ovarian and testicular degeneration and increased infant mortality are corollaries of too little manganese in the tissues.

Scientists believe inborn metabolism errors like maple syrup disease and PKU are related to a manganese deficiency. Disturbances in lipid and carbohydrate metabolism can also occur when body tissues are low in manganese. The trace element is involved in cholesterol synthesis; a deficiency can interrupt and even shut down the production of this substance. Decreased triglycerides and lipids, weight loss and intermittent nausea are other signs of manganese deficiency.

A deficiency can even cause transient dermatitis and a change in hair color to a reddish brown. A volunteer who consumed a diet deficient in manganese lost approximately 66 percent of his body manganese pool. He developed a prickly heat rash on his upper torso, groin and thighs. Serum cholesterol and high density lipoproteins plummeted, too.

Abnormalities of the pancreas can result in poor glucose utilization. This development suggests manganese may be involved with insulin formation.

Excessive intake of nutrients considered antagonistic to manganese also may contribute to a deficiency. Figures 28 and 29 list the vitamins and minerals that are antagonistic to manganese.

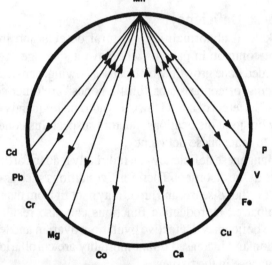

Figure 28
Minerals Antagonistic To Manganese

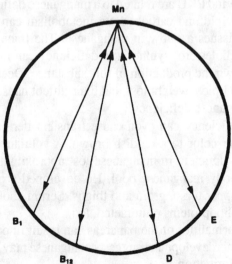

Figure 29
Vitamins Antagonistic To Manganese

A deficiency in trace elements that are synergistic can also lead to poor manganese status. Nutrients considered synergistic to manganese include the minerals iron, magnesium, phosphorus, potassium and zinc. The vitamins include A, B_1, B_3, B_5, B_6 and E.

Manganese Toxicity

Reports of manganese toxicity due to oral intake are relatively rare. Sufferers include those who have a chronic exposure to the substance in iron and steel factories, manganese ore mines, welding shops, chemical plants, dry cell battery factories, and petrochemical plants.

Physicians first discovered the problem in 1837, when mill workers began complaining of paralysis. In the 1930s doctors began focusing on manganese toxicity when miners began suffering the same symptoms.

There are three levels or grades of manganese toxicity. A manganese overload frequently causes degeneration of the neurons in various areas of the brain. Abnormalities in the neurotransmitters also can occur.

Mild toxicity symptoms include anorexia, insomnia, muscular pains, mental excitement, hallucinations, unaccountable laughter, impaired memory, and compulsive actions.

Moderate toxicity includes speech disorders, clumsy movements, abnormal gait, poor balance, hyperactive reflexes, and fine tremors.

Severe symptoms include rigidity, spasmodic laughter, and other symptoms similar to Parkinson's disease.

Alcoholics are more prone to manganese toxicity than others. So are people with iron deficiencies, chronic infections, kidney and bowel problems, which decrease its excretion.

Excessive manganese levels often are seen in conjunction with iron toxicity. In this case the manganese is not a toxin per se. Instead, its level rises because of the body's excessive iron retention. The manganese elevation may be due to the body's attempt to decrease the effects of iron toxicity. Or, the excess iron may be displacing manganese from storage tissues.

Excess manganese is suspected in tardive dyskinesia (TD), a disorder associated with abnormal movements, or twitches. TD is often associated with the use of an anti-psychotic drug, chlorpromazine, which apparently causes an increased accumulation of manganese in the brain. Manganese is also found elevated in individuals with hepatitis.

Manganese toxicity can be reduced by removing the exposure, e.g. changing jobs if you work in a high exposure plant. Adding antagonistic nutrients to the diet can also dissipate the toxicity if changing jobs is not an option. Figures 28 and 29 contain the trace elements antagonistic to manganese.

To date, there is no RDA for manganese. However, it has been reported that humans need a minimal intake of between 2.5 and 7 milligrams a day to meet the body's needs.

References

Kies, C., et al: Manganese Availability for Humans, Effect of Selected Dietary Factors. **Nutritional Bioavailability of Manganese.** Kies, C., Ed. Am.Chem.Soc. Wash., D.C., 1987.

Failla, M.L: Hormonal Regulation of Manganese. **Manganese in Metabolism and Enzyme Function.** Schrammk. V.L., Wedler, F.C., Eds. Academic Press. N.Y., 1986.

Leach, R.M. Jr: Metabolism and Function of Manganese. **Trace Elements in Human Health and Disease.** Vol.III. Prasad, A.S., Ed. Academic Press, N.Y. 1976.

Doisy, C.A. Jr: Micronutrient Control on Biosynthesis of Clotting Proteins and Cholesterol. **Trace Substances in Environmental Health,** VI. Hemphill, D.D., et al: Eds. Univ. Mo. Press. Columbia, Mo. 1973.

Strause, L., Saltmar, P: Role of Manganese in Bone Metabolism. **Nutritional Bioavailabilty of Manganese.** Kies, C., Ed. Am.Chem.Soc. Wash., D.C. 1987.

Keen, C.L., Lonnerdal, B: Manganese Toxicity in Man and Experimental Animals. **Manganese in Metabolism and Enzyme Function.** Schramm, V.L., Wedler, F.C., Eds. Academic Press. N.Y., 1986.

Weiner, W.J., et al: Effects of chlorpromazine on central nervous system concentrations of manganese, iron, and copper. **Life Sci.**, 20, 1971.

Chandra, S.V: Neurological Consequences of Manganese Imbalance. **Neurobiology of The Trace Elements,** Vol.2. Dreosti, I.E., Smith, R.M., Eds. Humana Press. N.J., 1983.

Aston, B.A: Manganese and Man. **J. Orthomol. Psych.** 9,4, 1980.

Chapter 11

Chromium

Mrs. G. was in a hurry to pick up her children from school when she made a left turn into a busy street. An unlicensed driver was speeding down the road and hit her traveling 30 miles per hour. The car spun and then crashed into a tree.

Mrs. G. was shook up but not seriously hurt, even though the car was totalled. But, for months afterward she would have frequent nightmares that recreated the accident. In a short period of time she developed diabetes — and a severe shortage of an important trace element called chromium.

When a stressful event occurs, the emotional changes in the body set up hormonal responses. These stressful life changes may create a glucose (blood sugar) intolerance, which can eventually lead to diabetes. People who have survived a severe car crash, plane crash or an ambush in a war, sometimes remain haunted by the incident for years. This continually affects their body chemistry. Their insulin and glucose levels may develop severe swings, which is a precursor to the development of diabetes.

Chromium Deficiency-Diabetes

Chromium works with insulin in allowing the cells to absorb and utilize glucose. Insulin is a hormone secreted by the pancreas that regulates carbohydrate metabolism and controls blood glucose levels. A deficiency of chromium has been found to produce increased insulin requirements.

Diabetes is caused by a number of factors. A series of related metabolic, endocrine, and nutritional disorders coalesce and cause the body to lose control of glucose and produce an abnormal amount of insulin. Since chromium and insulin work hand in hand, patients suffering from diabetes generally develop chromium deficiencies.

Peripheral Neuropathy

Peripheral neuropathy is characterized by numbness and tingling of the extremities that may be due to chromium deficiency. An example of this was reported in a patient who developed glucose intolerance, weight loss, peripheral neuropathy, and other metabolic disturbances. Increasing her insulin did not control the problems. However, when chromium was supplemented, her metabolic disturbances improved along with improvement in glucose control, as well as her neuropathy symptoms. Her insulin requirements were also eventually reduced with the addition of chromium.

Cardiovascular Heart Disease (CHD)

Studies have revealed that chromium is associated with the development of atherosclerosis. A deficiency of chromium has been found in individuals with high cholesterol levels and plaques in the aorta. Chromium supplementation has resulted in improvements in cholesterol levels and particularly the good cholesterol, high density lipoproteins, or (HDL).

Studies are showing that insulin itself may be the major contributing factor toward heart disease. Insulin levels have been found to be elevated in patients who have suffered heart attacks or who have clogged arteries. The effect of chromium in helping to reduce heart disease is due to its effect of improving insulin utilization and decreasing insulin requirements.

Hormonal Factors Contributing To Chromium Deficiency -Insulin

The hormone insulin contributes to chromium deficiency by increasing the excretion of the trace element. Patients with diabetes who receive insulin injections will tend to become deficient in chromium.

High refined sugar intake will also contribute to the loss of chromium as well as high blood sugar (glucose) levels. Eating foods with a high sugar content can make it very difficult for the body to maintain adequate chromium levels.

Estrogen

Chromium stores often become depleted during pregnancy. Pregnancy produces a state similar to diabetes that results in stepped up insulin secretion. It is likely that the hormone estrogen contributes to hyperinsulinism during pregnancy. Insulin levels are highest during the last trimester.

Women undergoing estrogen therapy may also begin to produce an excess of insulin, thus endangering the body's chromium stores.

Thyroid, Para-Thyroid

Thyroid activity may directly or indirectly affect one's chromium status. Insulin is known to decrease thyroid activity. Therefore, individuals with low thyroid activity have an increased requirement for chromium.

The para-thyroid when overactive, shares many of the symptoms of diabetes. One shared characteristic is excess insulin production, thus depleting chromium stores.

Tumors of the pancreas and pituitary gland may also cause insulin disturbances.

Stress

Physiological or emotional stress is known to affect chromium status of individuals. Physiological stress is a result of the body fighting off an infectious process for example. Patients who have suffered a heart attack commonly develop glucose intolerance. It has been proposed that a cardiac event can contribute to a diabetic condition.

Diabetic individuals suffering from emotional stress such as anxiety, depression, or other psychiatric conditions are known to have poor glucose control compared to diabetic patients without psychiatric symptoms.

It is obvious that emotional changes trigger hormonal responses. In clinical practice, doctors often see individuals who develop blood sugar problems following stressful or traumatic events, such as an automobile accident. An example of this was described previously. These patients may become emotionally stressed following the accident. Their insulin and glucose levels may develop severe swings, resulting in instability and poor response to therapy. This type of condition is called post traumatic dysinsulinism, a term meaning poor insulin control. The insulin level may be high one minute and very low an hour later. The hypo and hyperglycemic swings themselves can contribute to emotional stress. Therefore, abnormal insulin levels can contribute to mood swings ranging from depression to mania.

Factors Contributing To Chromium Deficiency - Dietary

Processing and refining remove a great deal of chromium from our foods. Losses are as high as 90 percent in some foods. Early studies compared the chromium content of the tissues of Americans to our European counterparts. Individuals in Europe had 2 to 12 times higher chromium levels than Americans. This was probably due to less refining of foods abroad. However, TMA studies of several thousand Europeans within the last two years do not show a major difference in TMA chromium levels. This is perhaps due to a similarity developing between the two continents, that is higher intake of refined carbohydrates.

Minerals

Figure 30 shows the minerals that are antagonistic to chromium and figure 31 shows the vitamins considered antagonistic to chromium. The solid lines indicate a direct antagonism either on a metabolic or absorption level. The broken lines indicate an indirect relationship. An individual with increased tissue retention of any one or combination of these elements can expect increased chromium requirements. Excess intake of these minerals can contribute to chromium losses or decreased absorption.

TRACE ELEMENTS and OTHER ESSENTIAL NUTRIENTS

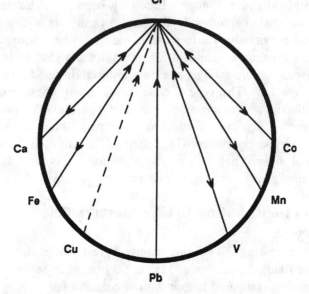

Figure 30
Minerals Antagonistic To Chromium

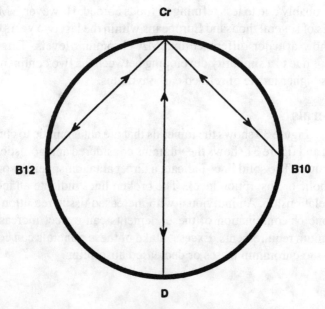

Figure 24
Vitamins Antagonistic To Chromium

The following minerals and vitamins are considered synergistic to chromium.

MINERALS SYNERGISTIC TO CHROMIUM	
Iron (Fe)	Manganese (Mn)
Magnesium (Mg)	Potassium (K)
Phosphorus (P)	Zinc (Zn)

VITAMINS SYNERGISTIC TO CHROMIUM	
Thiamin (B_1)	Vitamin A
Niacin (B_3)	Vitamin E
Riboflavin (B_2)	Pyridoxine (B_6)

Chromium Requirements

The total body content of chromium in an adult is about 6 milligrams. Tissue chromium levels are at their highest at birth and consequently decline with age.

The daily requirement for chromium is about one microgram per day. However, an individual should consume between 30 and 200 micrograms to fulfill that requirement due to the poor absorption of chromium.

Since chromium is known to spare protein and stabilize insulin, it can be an essential aid in weight control. Too much insulin production by the body or poor insulin utilization is commonly found with obesity. This is why most patients with adult onset diabetes are overweight. They are producing more than enough insulin, which has a fat storing effect.

Chromium also has been found useful in athletes, especially body builders. Due to the protein sparing effects, chromium improves the ability to build muscle size and lower body fat.

References

Mertz, W: Chromium Occurrence and Function in Biological Systems. **Physiol. Rev.** 49, 1969.

Wacker, W.E., Vallee, B.L: Chromium, Manganese, Iron, and other Metals in Ribonucleic Acid from Diverse Biological Sources. **J. Biol. Chem.** 234, 1959.

Anderson, et al: Urinary Chromium Excretion of Human Subjects: Effects of Chromium Supplementation and Glucose Loading. **Am. J. Clin. Nutr.** 36, 1982.

Doisy, R.J., et al: Chromium Metabolism in Man and Biochemical Effects. **Trace Elements in Human Health and Disease,** Vol. II. Prasad, A.S., Ed. Academic Press, N.Y., 1976.

Hunt, A.E., et al: Effect of Chromium Supplementation on Hair Chromium Concentration and Diabetic Status. **Fed. Proc.** 42, 1983.

Hambidge, K.M: Chromium Nutrition in Man. **Am. J. Clin. Nutr.** 27, 1974.

Hambidge, K.M., et al: The Concentration of Chromium in the Hair of Normal and Children with Juvenile Diabetes Mellitus. **Diabet.** 17, 1968.

Rosson, J.W., et al: Hair Chromium Concentrations in Adult Insulin Treated Diabetes. **Clin. Chim. Acta.** 93, 1979.

Jeejeebhoy, K.N., et al: Chromium Deficiency, Glucose Intolerance, and Neuropathy Reversed by Chromium Supplementation, in a Patient Receiving Long-Term Parenteral Nutrition. **Am. J. Clin. Nutr.** 30, 1977.

Schroeder, H.A., et al: Chromium Deficiency as a Factor in Atherosclerosis. **J. Chron. Dis.** 23, 1970.

Saner, G: **Chromium in Nutrition and Disease.** Alan R. Liss Inc., N.Y., 1980.

Stout, R.W: Insulin and Atheroma - An Update. **Lancet** I, 1987.

Mertz, W., et al: Relation of Chromium Excretion to Glucose Metabolism in Human Subjects. **Fed. Proc.** 36, 1977.

Mertz, W: Chromium and its Relationship to Carbohydrate Metabolism. **The Medical Clinics of North America,** Vol 60. W.B.Saunders Co., Phil. 1976.

Hambidge, K.M., Rodgerson, D.O: Comparison of Hair Chromium Levels of Nulliparous and Parous Women. **Am. J. Ob. Gyn.** 103, 1969.

Felig, P: Body Fuel Metabolism and Diabetes Mellitus in Pregnancy. **The Medical Clinics of North America.,** Vol. 61. W.B. Saunders, Co., Phil., 1977.

Spellacy, W.N., Goetz, F.C: Plasma Insulin in Normal and Late Pregnancy. **N.E.J.M.,** 268, 1963.

Gershberg, H., et al: Glucose Tolerance in Women Receiving an Ovulatory Suppressant. **Diabet.** 13, 1964.

Javier, A., et al: Ovulatory Suppressants, Estrogen, and Carbohydrate Metabolism. **Metbol.** 17, 1968.

Gray, R.S., et al: Hypercholesterolemia in Diabetics with Clinically Unrecognized Primary Thyroid Failure. **Horm. Metab. Res.** 13, 1981.

Husband, D.J., Alberti, K: "Stress" hyperglycemia During Acute Myocardial Infarction: An Indication of Pre-Existing Diabetes. **Lancet,** Jul., 1983.

Lusterman, P.J., et al: Stress and Diabetic Control. **Lancet,** Mar., 1983.

Mooradian, A.D., Morley, J.E: Micronutrient Status in Diabetes Mellitus. **Am. J. Clin. Nutr.** 45,5, 1987.

Leclerq-Meyer, V., et al: Effect of Calcium and Magnesium on Glucagon Secretion. **Endocrinol.,** 93, 1977.

Vitamin D and Insulin Secretion. **Nutr. Rev.,** 44,11, 1986.

Chapter 12

Selenium

Selenium was discovered by Berzelius in 1817 and was named after the moon. Eventually the electrical and optical properties of selenium were recognized and stimulated a great deal of research and development in the electrophotographic field. This led to the use of selenium in the xerographic or photocopy processes.

Initially there was little biological interest in the mineral selenium except for its toxic properties. Selenium toxicity was first recognized and described in animals. Cattle grazing on certain plants grown in high selenium soil developed a peculiar condition called alkali disease or blind staggers, that eventually leads to death. It was believed that humans living in the same regions could also be affected by too much selenium. However, toxicity in humans was not readily recognized.

Interest in selenium increased due to the discovery of a selenium compound called "factor 3." This compound was found to protect animals from fatty infiltration and necrosis of the liver. This also led to the speculation that some type of relationship existed between selenium and vitamin E. Research by Schwarz and Foltz, at the National Institutes of Health in 1957, found that selenium deficiency produced recognizable abnormalities in lab animals. They found that selenium supplementation reversed a condition called white muscle disease that occurred in sheep and cattle raised on selenium deficient soils. This led to the suspicion that selenium may be involved as a cofactor in enzyme systems related to cellular oxidation, and that selenium may play a role in human nutrition as well. The discovery that selenium deficiency was related to disease conditions brought selenium to the forefront as one of the latest essential nutrients.

The research of Rotruck and colleagues found that a deficiency of selenium resulted in oxidative damage to red blood cells, which was related to reduced activity of an enzyme, glutathione peroxidase. This enzyme reduced the effects of hydrogen peroxide upon hemoglobin. Eventually it was found that selenium was a component of the glutathione peroxidase enzyme, which establishes a direct biochemical role for selenium.

Selenium Toxicity And Deficiency In Animals

The effect of selenium toxicity and deficiency have been well described in animals, and vary according to species. Selenium toxicity or selenosis occurs mostly in ruminants or grazing animals due to the consumption of selenium accumulating plants, such as locoweed. These plants preferentially accumulate selenium when the mineral is present in the soil in high concentrations. The accumulator plants can convert inorganic selenium into a utilizable form. However, after these plants die, the organic form of selenium is returned to the soil and can then be utilized by other plants as well. Areas of high selenium soil are found in the North American plains, Wyoming, South Dakota, Nebraska, and Oregon. Other countries known to have high selenium areas include Australia, Israel, Ireland, South Africa, South America, the former Soviet Union, France, Germany, and China. Symptoms of toxicity that have been described include:

ACUTE SELENIUM TOXICITY SYMPTOMS IN ANIMALS	
Abdominal pains	Blindness
Excessive salivation	Partial paralysis
Respiratory distress	Starvation

CHRONIC SELENIUM TOXICITY SYMPTOMS IN ANIMALS	
Rough coats	Hair loss
Lameness	Pain and sloughing of hooves
Erosion of joints	Cardiac Atrophy
Liver cirrhosis	Anemia (in all species)
Lowered conception rates	Birth defects

The mechanism of selenium toxicity remains uncertain. However, it may be due to the effects of excess selenium inhibiting enzymes and proteins essential to normal cellular processes. Antagonism of other nutrients by selenium may also play a significant role in selenium toxicity.

Selenium is necessary for reproduction and growth in animals and is known to protect against a number of diseases. Conditions such as white muscle disease, exudative diathesis, pancreatic fibrosis, and liver disease are prevented by adequate selenium in various species. These conditions have been related to excessive free radical formation and reduced glutathione peroxidase activity.

Selenium In Human Nutrition - Deficiency

The most recognized condition associated with selenium deficiency in humans is Keshan disease, a cardiomyopathy that affects mostly children and young women. Keshan disease was discovered in China in people living in areas where selenium was very low in the soil. Their major food staple was grains and cereals that contained little, if any, selenium. The hair and blood selenium levels of these people were very low and they improved only after being supplemented with selenium.

Kashin-Beck disease is also found in individuals living in low selenium areas. Kashin-Beck is an osteoarthritic condition affecting children in their developmental years. It is also known as "big-joint" disease due to swelling and calcium deposition in affected joints. However, it is believed that selenium deficiency alone is not the sole cause of these conditions.

Prasad has reviewed a number of conditions that may be related to selenium deficiency. These are summarized below.

Cataracts

Selenium concentrations normally increase in the human lens from birth to old age. However, the selenium content of lenses with cataracts was found to be markedly reduced, less than one sixth, compared to normal lenses in the same age group. Glutathione, the selenium dependent enzyme is also present in high amounts in normal lenses compared to those with cataracts. Any factor that antagonizes selenium or the selenium-dependent enzyme system, can allow oxidative damage to occur. Some drugs, due to their production of excessive free radicals during their metabolism, are known to cause cataracts. Therefore, xenobiotics, drugs, and heavy metals such as mercury, can contribute to cataract formation, especially when selenium is deficient.

Red Blood Cell (Erythrocyte) Disorders

Hemolytic anemia, as well as simple iron deficiency anemia, has been associated with selenium deficiency due to reduced glutathione peroxidase activity. A decrease in this selenium-dependent enzyme glutathione peroxidase has been reported in normal and premature infants and in those with jaundice. Glanzmann's disease, a platelet disorder characterized by excessive bleeding due to poor clotting, is associated with reduced glutathione peroxidase activity.

Schrauzer also reviewed studies associated with selenium deficiency which are discussed below.

Aging

During normal metabolism, free radicals are produced. It is estimated that each cell is subject to approximately one thousands "oxidative hits" per day. This is normal and is thought to contribute to the normal aging process. However, excessive free radical production or a reduced ability to quench the normal production of radicals is thought to contribute to premature or accelerated aging. Selenium deficiency has been associated with degenerative conditions of aging due to decreased glutathione peroxidase activity. These include premature aging, lipofuscin deposition, and chronic inflammatory conditions.

Cancer

Experimental studies have demonstrated a protective effect of selenium on mammary tumor formation and reduced tumor growth rates in animals. Selenium deficiency, in conjunction with low vitamin E, has been related to a greater incidence of lung, skin, and gastrointestinal cancers in humans. Selenium protects against chromosomal damage, stimulates DNA repair, and modulates the rate of cell division. Selenium also has an inhibitory effect upon chemical carcinogens and accelerates their detoxification.

Immune Competence

Selenium, in conjunction with vitamin E, enhances antibody formation. Therefore, selenium deficiency may impair the normal immune response. Studies have revealed low selenium status in AIDS patients, and selenium deficiencyhas been associated with progression of the disease. There are similarities between AIDS cardiomyopathy and cardiomyopathy found in Keshan disease. Reports have indicated improvements in AIDS related cardiomyopathy as result of selenium therapy.

Sudden Infant Death Syndrome (SIDS)

A commentary by Oldfield cited studies associating selenium deficiency with (SIDS). This remains controversial at this time however.

Cystic Fibrosis

Oldfield also cited studies speculating the relationship between selenium deficiency and cystic fibrosis. Wallach has shown convincing evidence of this relationship. He reported a direct relationship of cystic fibrosis in the rhesus monkey with selenium and zinc deficiency. Wallach relates a strong indirect relationship to cystic fibrosis in humans and selenium deficiency in conjunction with deficiencies of vitamin E and zinc. Liver analysis of selenium in children with cystic fibrosis showed a significant reduction of selenium compared to normal children.

Crohn's Disease

A study of patients with Crohn's disease found that a reduction of selenium and glutathione peroxidase in plasma and erythrocytes existed in 40 percent of an affected group. They also found that patients with bowel resections of 200 centimeters or more were at a high risk for developing selenium deficiency due to malabsorption.

Thyroid

Selenium has been shown to be related to thyroid function. The enzyme 1 iodothyronine deiodinase (IDI) is a selenoenzyme, which is responsible for the peripheral conversion of T4 to T3 in the liver and kidneys. IDI activity is reduced in the presence of selenium deficiency.

Factors Contributing To Selenium Deficiency

There are several factors that can contribute to selenium deficiency other than reduced intake. Figure 32 shows the minerals that are antagonistic to selenium. The solid lines represent the known antagonism, and the broken lines indicate suspected antagonism.

Sulfur (S) protects from selenium toxicity. However, large amounts of selenium can interfere with normal sulfur metabolism.

The antagonistic effects between selenium and silver (Ag), arsenic (As), cadmium (Cd), mercury (Hg), and thallium (Tl) have been described by Ganther. It should be noted that selenium does protect tissues from the toxic effects of heavy metals, but excretions of toxic heavy metals are not increased by selenium therapy. Selenium apparently binds these metals, such as mercury and cadmium, rendering them less damaging to cells and tissues.

Fluorine (F) has been shown to counteract the effects of selenosis. This has been found in areas with high levels of both selenium and fluorine. Selenium was not toxic even with a high body burden when fluorine was also present.

Antagonism of lead (Pb), tin (Sn), and zinc (Zn) has been cited by Schrauzer. More recent investigations have confirmed the zinc-selenium antagonism. Copper (Cu) has also been shown to be a selenium antagonist.

On the basis of TMA studies it is suspected that selenium is antagonistic to magnesium. This is due to the potential sodium raising effect of selenium. Sodium increases the excretion of magnesium. Magnesium is also essential for the synthesis of glutathione, and a deficiency of magnesium can increase the effects of selenium toxicity.

The possibility of iron and manganese antagonism by selenium also exists. Anemia is a consistent finding in animals and humans with selenium toxicity.

Figure 32
Minerals Antagonistic To Selenium

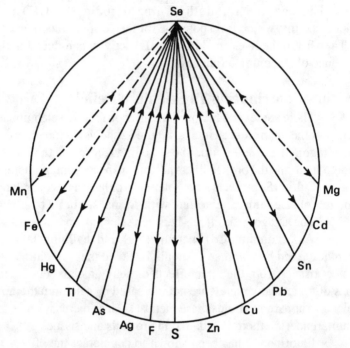

Figure 33 illustrates the vitamins that are considered antagonistic to selenium. Animals suffering from selenosis were found to have decreased levels of vitamin A and ascorbic acid. Ip reported that the protective effect of selenium on mammary carcinoma in animals was nullified by high vitamin C supplementation. Selenium toxicity in laboratory animals is associated with a corresponding decrease in the levels of vitamin C, and vitamin K.

The nutrients shown in figure 32 and 33 can be antagonized by excessive selenium accumulation. They, in turn, can inhibit the toxic effects of too much selenium.

Figure 33
Vitamins Antagonistic To Selenium

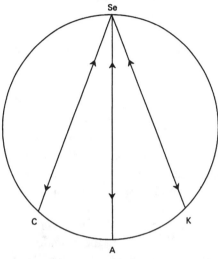

Nutrients Synergistic To Selenium

Vitamin E is well recognized as a selenium co-factor or synergist. Vitamin E is a fat soluble vitamin that acts as an antioxidant and protects the lipid cell membranes from the effects of oxidation. Vitamin E supplementation can reduce the symptoms of selenium deficiency.

Cobalt (Co) has also been shown to be synergistic to selenium. A diet containing high amounts of selenium did not produce selenium toxicity symptoms in lab animals initially. However, when cobalt was added in equal amounts, symptoms of selenosis developed.

Vitamin B_6 acts as a selenium synergist and is associated with the conversion of selenomethionine to glutathione peroxidase.

Even though in some circumstances vitamin C can antagonize selenium, in others it can enhance selenium utilization. Human studies have revealed that vitamin C plays a role in the maintenance of selenium homeostasis.

Copper has also been shown to be synergistic to selenium. Animal studies have revealed that glutathione peroxidase activity decreased during copper deficiency.

Human Selenium Toxicity

Selenium has been recognized as a toxin for many years before it was determined to be a required nutrient. Toxicity symptoms have been extensively studied and reported in high selenium areas of China. Toxicity has since been reported in the United States and other countries.

Sources Of Selenium

Selenium intoxication has been caused by industrial exposure for decades. Fishbein has categorized the primary and secondary industrial exposures to selenium. Primary industries include mining, ore extraction, including copper, zinc, lead, pyrite roasting, and the production of lime, and cement. These industries expose workers to various types of selenium containing dusts. Secondary sources produce organic vapors and fumes containing selenium compounds that include the manufacture of glass and ceramics, steel and brass production. Vulcanizing and curing of rubber products release organic selenium vapors. Selenium is a potential hazard in the plastic and electronic industry and is contained in paint pigments and printing inks. Chiau and colleague cited reports of high selenium concentrations in paper products, which when burned, give off a significant amount of selenium. These levels are high enough to be considered toxic.

Selenium intoxication has been found in individuals taking nutritional supplements. The supplements contained much more selenium than the amounts listed on the labels. The average selenium intake of individuals affected by selenium toxicity in high selenium water and soil areas of China was approximately 5 milligrams per day.

Symptoms Of Selenium Toxicity

The signs and symptoms of selenium toxicity have been described by several investigators, and even though the sources vary, the symptoms are very similar. Symptoms of industrial exposure have been described by Fishbein, depending upon the type of selenium the workers were exposed to. Acute exposure produced irritation of the eyes, nose, and throat, burning sensation of the nostrils, sneezing, coughing, congestion, and dizziness.

Dyspnea, headaches, and edema of the uvula were found with heavy exposures. Chronic exposure has produced hypochromic anemia, leukopenia, irregular menses, and a garlic breath odor, or metallic taste.

Symptoms associated with excessive ingestion of selenium from supplements described by Levander and Burk include nausea, vomiting, hair loss, changes in the nails, fatigue, irritability, and peripheral neuropathy.

Changes occurring in individuals living in high selenium soil areas include nausea, vomiting, skin depigmentation, hair loss, and low hemoglobin. Dental caries has been a consistent finding in regions of selenosis. The effect of selenium on the teeth has been confirmed by animal studies.

A case of selenium toxicity was reported with the use of a selenium-containing anti-dandruff shampoo when skin lesions were present. The selenium was readily absorbed through the open skin. Symptoms included tremors and appetite loss, which improved with discontinuation of the product.

Interestingly, the topical application of selenomethionine has proven beneficial in protecting against skin cancer caused by ultraviolet irradiation.

Sources Of Selenium And Body Distribution

The selenium content of cereals and grains are considered good sources of the mineral. However, the content would vary depending upon the amount of selenium present in the soil in which the crops were grown, as well as the preparation methods. Seafood, kidney, liver, meats, and poultry are also good sources. Fruits and vegetables, except for garlic and asparagus, are poor sources of selenium.

Selenium is distributed throughout the body with the highest concentrations found in the kidneys and liver. Whole body selenium content has been estimated at 3 - 6 milligrams in individuals living in low selenium areas and approximately 13 milligrams in other regions.

A U.S. recommended daily allowance for selenium has not been established. However, a safe and adequate daily intake has been estimated to be 50 to 200 micrograms for adults and children above the age of 7. This range has been extrapolated from animal studies. It is estimated that Americans and Canadians consume between 62 and 216 micrograms in their daily diet. Canadians apparently have a higher intake than Americans. This is also apparent from the hair tissue mineral analysis (TMA) studies conducted by this laboratory on individuals living in different countries. The information is depicted in the following table.

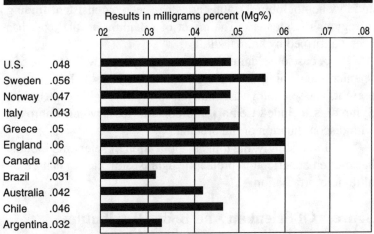

Table 3

HAIR SELENIUM LEVELS OF POPULATION GROUPS FROM VARIOUS COUNTRIES.

Country	Mg%
U.S.	.048
Sweden	.056
Norway	.047
Italy	.043
Greece	.05
England	.06
Canada	.06
Brazil	.031
Australia	.042
Chile	.046
Argentina	.032

Note: These values are averages, based upon multiple samples from each country. Tests were performed by the procedures established by Trace Elements, Inc.

Assessment Of Selenium Status

The mean concentration of selenium in whole blood was found to be 20.6 ug/100ml in a U.S. population. The range was 10-34 ug/100ml. Similar findings were reported in a Canadian population. The findings did range somewhat to the local distribution of selenium in the soil and water.

Selenium status has also been reported in disease conditions. Children suffering from kwashiorkor, a protein deficiency due to starvation, had a mean level of 11 ug/100ml compared to 23 ug in control groups. A reduction has also been noted in burn patients. Other conditions associated with low selenium include alcoholic cirrhosis, cancers, muscular complaints, hypertension, atherosclerosis, arthritis, muscular dystrophy, infertility, macular degeneration, and diabetic neuropathy.

The use of plasma or erythrocyte glutathione peroxidase has been found useful in evaluating selenium deficiency. However, analysis of this selenium-dependent enzyme, although excellent for determining a deficiency is not sufficient for monitoring adequate or toxic levels.

Tissue mineral analysis (TMA) of the hair has been used in the study of Keshan disease, and researchers have shown that the blood and hair selenium levels are closely related. TMA is very useful in evaluating selenium in relationship to the other antagonistic and synergistic mineral co-factors.

Conclusion

Even though the interest in selenium in the nutritional field has increased, there is still a great deal to be learned about this important trace element. The focus of selenium research has been on its involvement in the anti-oxidant system. However, its biological involvement may be far more extensive.

As with any nutrient, selenium should not be viewed in isolation. A deficiency or excess of selenium will have an impact on several other nutrients. Therefore, assessment of an individual's selenium status should be made in conjunction with its antagonists, synergists, and other co-factors.

References

McLester JS: **Nutrition and diet in health and disease 4th Ed.** WB Saunders, Phil. 128-129, 1943.

Williams SR: **Nutrition and diet therapy 2nd Ed.** Mosby, St Louis. 150, 1973.

Rotruck JT, Pope AL, Ganther HE, Swanson AB, Hateman DG, Hoekstra WG: Selenium: Biochemical role as a component of glutathione peroxidase. **Science** 179:588-590, 1973.

Underwood EJ: **Trace elements in human and animal nutrition.** Academic Press, NY. 302-340, 1977.

Yang G, Ge K, Chen J, Chen X: Selenium related endemic diseases and the daily selenium requirement of humans. **World Nutr. Rev. Diet.** 55:98-152, 1988.

Yang G, et al: The role of selenium in Keshan disease. **Adv. Nutr. Res.** 6:203-231, 1984.

Prasad AS: **Trace elements and iron in human metabolism.** Plenum Pub. NY. 215-250, 1978.

Schrauzer GN: Selenium in nutritional cancer prophylaxis: An update. **Vitamins, nutrition, and cancer**. Prasad AS, Ed. Karger Pub. Basel. 240-250, 1984.

Chandra RK: **Immunology of nutritional disorders**. Year Book Med. Pub. Chicago. 54, 1980.

Cirelli A, et al: Serum selenium concentration and disease progress in patients with HIV infection. **Clin. Biochem.** 24:211-214, 1991.

Dworkin BM, et al: Selenium deficiency in the acquired immunodeficiency syndrome. **J. Parenteral and Ent. Nutr.** 10:405-407, 1986.

Oldfield JE: The two faces of selenium. **J. Nutr.** 117:2002-2008, 1987.

Wallach JD: Cystic fibrosis: A proposal of etiology and pathogenesis. **Quantum Med**. 1.2:1-48, 1988.

Rannem T, et al: Selenium status in patients with Crohn's disease. **Am. J. Clin. Nutr**. 56:933-937, 1992.

Aaseth J, Aadland E, Thomassen Y: Serum selenium in patients with short bowel syndrome. **Selenium in biology and medicine part B**. Combs, Spallholz, Levander, Oldfield, Eds. AVI, NY. 976-980, 1987.

Essential trace elements and thyroid hormones. **Lancet** 339:1575, 1992.

Goodhart RS, Shils ME: **Modern nutrition in health and disease**. Lea and Fediger, Phil. 392-393, 1976.

Ganther HE: Biochemistry of selenium. **Selenium**. Zingaro, Cooper, Eds. VNR, NY. 546-614, 1974.

Bian-Sheng L, Shen-Si L: Endemic selenosis and fluorosis. **Selenium in biology and medicine part B.** Combs, Spallholz, Levander, Oldfield, Eds. AVI, NY. 708-711, 1987.

House WA, Welch RM: Bioavailability of and interactions between zinc and silver in rats fed wheat grain intrinsically labeled with zinc and selenium. **J. Nutr.** 119:916-921, 1989.

Jensen L: Modification of a selenium toxicity in chicks by dietary silver and copper. **J. Nutr.** 105:769, 1975.

Minnich V, et al: Glutathione biosynthesis in human erythrocytes. Identification of the enzymes of glutathione synthesis in hemolysates. **J. Clin. Invest.** 50:507-513, 1971.

Yan L, Boylan M, Spallholz, JE: Effect of dietary selenium and magnesium on human mammary tumor growth in athymic nude mice. **Nut. Cancer** 16:239-248, 1991.

Fishbein L: Toxicology of selenium and tellurium. **Toxicology of trace elements.** Goyer, Mehlman, Eds. John Wiley, NY. 191-240, 1977.

Ip C: Susceptibility of mammary carcinogenesis in response to dietary selenium levels: Modifications by fat and vitamin intake. **Selenium in biology and medicine part B.** *Combs,* et al Eds. VNR, NY. 664 674, 1974.

Cooper CW, Glover JR: The toxicology of selenium and its compounds. **Selenium.** Zingaro, Cooper, Eds. VNR, NY. 664-674, 1974.

Kirchgessner M, Schwarz FJ, Schnegg A: Interactions of essential metals in human physiology. **Clinical biochemical, and nutritional aspects of trace elements.** Prasad AS, Ed. AR Liss, NY. 472-512, 1982.

Beilstein MA, Whanger PD: Effects of vitamin B-6 deficiency on selenium metabolism in the rat. **J. Nutr.** 119:1962-1972, 1989.

Martin RF, et al: Ascorbic acid-selenite interactions in humans studies with an oral dose of $^{74}SeO_3^{2-}$ **Am J. Clin. Nutr.** 49:862-869, 1989.

Vitamin C can promote selenium utilization. **Nutr. Rev.** 48:290-291, 1990.

L'abbe MR, Fischer PWF, Chavez ER: Changes in selenium and antioxidant status during DMBA-induced mammary carcinogenesis in rats. **J. Nutr.** 119:766-771, 1989.

Zidenberg-Cherr S, Keen CL: Essential trace elements in antioxidant processes. **Trace elements, micronutrients, and free radicals.** Dreosti JE, Ed. Humana Press, NJ. 107-127, 1991.

Yang GQ, Wang S, Zhou R, Sun S: Endemic selenium intoxication of humans in China. **Am. J. Clin. Nutr.** 37:872-881.

Chiou KY, Manuel OK: Emission of Chalcogen elements in air. **Trace substances in environmental health XIX.** Hemphill DD, Ed. Univ. Mo. Columbia. 556-66, 1985.

Levander OA, Burk RF: Selenium. **Present knowledge in nutrition 6th ed.** Brown ML, Ed. Int. Life Sci. Found. Wash. DC. 268-273, 1990.

Burke RF: Selenium in man. **Trace elements in human health and disease vol. II.** Prasad, Oberleas, Eds. Academic Press, NY. 105-133, 1976.

Underwood EJ: **Trace elements in human and animal nutrition 4th ed.** Academic Press, NY. 339-340, 1977.

Ransone JW, Scott NM, Koblock EC: Selenium sulfide intoxication. **N.E.J.M.** 264:384-385, 1961.

Burke KE, et al: The effects of topical and oral l-selenomethionine on pigmentation and skin cancer cancer induced by ultraviolet irradiation. **Nutr. Cancer,** 17:123-137, 1992.

Bennet BG, Peterson PJ: Assessment of human exposure to environmental selenium. **Selenium in biology and medicine part B.** Combs, et al, Eds. 608-618, 1987.

National Research Council, Food and Nutrition Board. Committee on dietary allowances. **Recommended daily allowance 9th ed.** Nat Acad. Sci. Wash. 185, 1980.

Levander OA: Selenium: Biochemical action, interactions and some human health implications. **Clinical, biochemical and nutritional aspects of trace elements.** Prasad AS, Ed. AR Liss, NY. 345-368, 1982.

Ganther HE: Biochemistry of selenium. **Selenium.** Zingaro RA, Cooper WC, Eds. VNR, NY. 546-614, 1974.

Prasad AS: **Trace elements and iron in human metabolism.** Plenum Pub., NY. 234, 1978.

Robinson MF: Clinical effects of selenium deficiency and excess. **Clinical, biochemical and nutritional aspects of trace elements.** Prasad AS, Ed. AR Liss, NY. 325-343, 1982.

Chapter 13

Sodium, Potassium, Chloride

Sodium and potassium are frequently referred to as electrolytes, since they carry a positive electrical charge (cation) in the fluids of the body. The abundance of sodium is concentrated in the extracellular fluids and potassium is found largely inside the the cells. The difference in concentration provides an electrical potential across cell membranes. This electrical potential is particularly important and necessary for nerve conduction, muscle contraction, fluid balance, and acid-alkali balance. Chloride carries a negative charge (anion) and is the major extracellular negatively charged ion. Chloride helps in maintaining a charge difference when sodium and potassium move back and forth across cell membranes. Chloride also activates salivary amylase and is removed from the blood by the parietal cells of the stomach for the production of hydrochloric acid. Maintenance of sodium, potassium and chloride in their respective locations is controlled by a series of enzymatic reactions called ionic pumps and specific channels in cell membranes. These channels are very specific and only allow their specific mineral through the cell membrane. Therefore, each cell has sodium channels, potassium channels, calcium channels, etc.

Requirements

The intake of chloride parallels sodium in the form of sodium chloride. The Food and Nutrition Board have determined the following estimates of safe and adequate daily sodium intake: Infants 0-6 months, 115-350 milligrams (mg)., children 6 months to 1 year, 250-750 mg., children 1-3 years, 325-975, 4-6 years, 450-1350 mg., 7-10 years 600-1800 mg., 11 years and older 900-2700 mg., adults 1100-3300 mg. During pregnancy an additional 69 mg. per day is the estimated average requirement.

The minimum requirement for potassium is estimated at 1600-2000 milligrams per day, depending upon the diet. For example, a total vegetarian eating mainly fruits and vegetables may consume 8,000 to 11,000 milligrams of potassium per day. The average intake on a typical non-vegetarian diet is about 2,500 milligrams per day.

Regulation

Sodium is regulated by a number of factors including behavioral, physiological, psychological, neurological and hormonal. Plasma and tissue levels are maintained closely, even though the intake can vary widely from day to day and under many different circumstances. The kidneys are the main regulator of these electrolytes. When sodium is low, due to low intake or excessive loss from the body, the kidneys will respond by conserving the mineral. When intake is high, the kidneys will allow more to be excreted. Sodium is conserved or retained through reabsorption by the kidneys and potassium by regulation of its secretion. Sodium can effect potassium balance, and potassium can in turn effect sodium regulation by the kidneys. For example, if an excessive amount of potassium develops, more sodium will be reabsorbed by the kidneys and more potassium will be secreted. If sodium becomes excessive, then the kidneys will allow less sodium reabsorption and decrease potassium secretion. This is accomplished through a series of hormonal and physiological reactions.

Renin is a hormone formed by the small blood vessels in the kidneys. When released into the blood stream it acts upon other enzymes that eventually result in the formation of angiotensin. Angiotensin then acts upon the adrenal cortex, causing it to increase the rate of production of a hormone called aldosterone. Aldosterone is the major hormone affecting sodium retention. When sodium levels are low in the body, aldosterone production increases, causing the kidneys to conserve sodium. This hormone also causes salt hunger, or a craving for a salty substance. Salt craving is also caused by adrenal corticotrophic hormone (ACTH) secreted from the pituitary gland. When sodium levels are normal or high, aldosterone levels decrease, resulting in less sodium reabsorption by the kidneys.

Water balance is affected by sodium, potassium, and chloride status as well as the mechanism that control them. When dehydration occurs, either intracellular or extracellular dehydration, an antidiuretic hormone (ADH) is produced that stimulates water conservation. ADH is actually responsible for thirst. Dehydration affects the concentrations of sodium, potassium and chloride. When there is an increase in the concentration of sodium, the body responds by increasing our thirst. Water is consumed, the kidneys increase the reabsorption of water and the concentration is normalized.

The sympathetic nervous system also plays a major role in regulating sodium and chloride. Stimulation of the sympathetic nervous system during periods of stress causes an increase in sodium retention. When sodium concentrations are low, the sympathetic system will "kick in" in order to improve the body's sodium level.

Physiological changes will increase sodium hunger and intake. Excessive perspiration due to working in hot climates or strenuous excerise increase the body's electrolyte needs. During pregnancy sodium requirements increase as well. This is due to excessive losses that occur during pregnancy and are caused by an increase in hormones such as estrogen, progesterone, oxytocin, and prolactin.

Principle hormones that affect the cellular uptake of potassium include insulin and epinephrine.

Deficiency

Electrolyte deficiencies in the blood serum and dehydration can arise from kidney disease, prolonged diarrhea, excessive vomiting, profuse sweating, laxative abuse, adrenal insufficiency, and hypothyroidism. Serum potassium deficiency can develop due to increased accumulation of intracellular potassium. This can be caused by a shift in the acid-alkali balance. When the plasma becomes too alkaline, potassium moves from the plasma into the cells. Protein and other nutritional deficiencies are also associated with potassium and sodium loss. Hormonal imbalances and some drugs can contribute to fluid and electrolyte imbalances.

Addison's disease is a condition caused by the inability of the adrenal glands to produce adequate amounts of the sodium retaining hormones.

Sodium deficiency or hyponatriemia can cause symptoms of headaches, confusion, seizures and coma. Mild hypokalemia or potassium deficiency can result in fatigue, weakness, muscle cramping and heart arrhythmia. More severe deficiencies can result in paralysis and death.

Excesses

Excessive sodium retention (hypernatremia) can develop as a result of excessive intake. Hypernatremia can also develop due to a greater loss of water from the body relative to sodium, even without excessive sodium intake. Increased adrenal production of aldosterone can contribute to hypernatremia, as well as heavy metals such as cadmium, or various vitamin and mineral imbalances. Sodium excess is associated with restlessness, irritability and lethargy. Seizures and death can occur with very high levels.

Hyperkalemia can result from the movement of potassium from intracellular compartments to the extracellular fluid. This can be caused by acidosis, kidney disease, strenuous exercise, and overdose of drugs such as digitalis. Hyperkalemia can produce neurological disturbances such as numbness of the hands and feet, cardiac arrhythmia and paralysis.

Hypertension

Several years ago the U.S. government issued warnings to the entire population that eating salt increased the risk of high blood pressure. This warning was based upon studies of primitive cultures who had a very low dietary salt intake and who also did not have a prevalence of high blood pressure. The research concluded that salt must be the cause of hypertension in people living in industrialized countries. As a result, many people began stringently reducing their salt intake for themselves and their families. Salt was soon to become known as the "silent killer." Advertisements and commercials advocated the reduction of salt intake for life. Eventually low salt and no-salt foods appeared on every grocery shelf

It now appears that the salt-hypertension link was overly exaggerated. In fact, stringent salt restriction is only necessary for a small segment of the affected population. Only about 10-15 percent may benefit from limiting salt intake. These are a group individuals with high blood pressure who are classified as "salt-sensitive." For this group, restricting salt intake may help to keep their blood pressure from going higher. This, however, does not mean that eating salt causes high blood pressure. The Intersalt study compared 52 groups of people in 32 different countries and concluded that salt intake does not matter much. There was apparently little relationship between salt consumption and blood pressure.

More recent studies implicate chloride in the development of hypertension rather than sodium alone. Animal studies have shown that high amounts of sodium chloride can induce an elevation in blood pressure, which did not occur when equal amounts of sodium bicarbonate were given. Blood pressure elevation even occurred with high intake of potassium chloride.

It becomes evident in light of the above information that sodium chloride alone is not the major culprit in the development of hypertension. However, individual susceptibility is a more important factor. As mentioned previously, some individuals are considered sodium-sensitive or perhaps more appropriately "chloride-sensitive." Another large segment of the population, however, may be considered sodium-insensitive and have a reduced ability to retain sodium, even though their sodium intake may be high. This brings us back to the recognition of metabolic individuality, and that a general recommendation of sodium restriction may not be appropriate.

Factors Contributing To Sodium Chloride Sensitivity

In earlier chapters we discussed the fact that diet is not controlled by just what we consume. The neuro-endocrine system is the major player in our nutritional status. This is why some individuals can take in an abundance of sodium chloride and yet retain little of what they consume. On the other hand, some individuals consume very little sodium and yet retain much more than others. These are the fast metabolic types who tend to retain sodium like a sponge retains water. The fast metabolic type has an elevated metabolic rate due to an increased sympathetic neuro-endocrine system. The sympathetic nervous system, as well as the adrenal and thyroid glands, are overactive and contribute to the increased retention of sodium. This pattern is associated with the "type A" personality and is readily aggravated by stress. A University of North Carolina study showed that a group of students when subjected to psychological stress in a "quiz show" atmosphere had increased retention of fluids as well as sodium. The group of students who had this response were from what was considered a high risk group: one or both parents had a history of hypertension. Fast metabolic types would be considered sodium-sensitive since they have such a strong tendency to retain sodium, even if their intake is low.

Other nutritional factors can be involved in sodium chloride sensitivity. For example, cadmium, a toxic heavy metal, will cause sodium retention due to its effect upon the kidneys. Nutritional minerals in excess such as iron, selenium, and nickel can increase the tendency to retain sodium. Deficiency of calcium, magnesium and potassium can also contribute to increased sodium retention. When magnesium becomes deficient in the body, the sodium retaining hormones produced by the adrenal glands increase in production and/or become more dominant, adding to the problem of increased sodium retention. These nutrients in turn can be used in combatting the effects of sodium retention. Magnesium intake can reduce the adrenal cortical hyperfunctioning and has been shown to help control high blood pressure. Potassium is antagonistic to sodium and can reduce sodium-sensitive hypertension. Calcium increases the excretion of sodium and decreases sympathetic neurological activity and has also been found to reduce hypertension.

Studies have shown that in hypertensive and non-hypertensive groups the amount of sodium chloride intake is very similar. However, the calcium intake was notably different. The normotensive group consumed about 400 milligrams of calcium per day while hypertensive groups consume much less, about 140 milligrams. It is probably no coincidence that the average calcium intake is far below acceptable levels in the population considered to be at risk for the development of high blood pressure: Afro-Americans and the elderly.

Sodium, Potassium And TMA Studies

Generally speaking, TMA sodium and potassium levels indicate adrenal status. Usually when sodium is elevated, potassium is also elevated. When sodium is lower than normal, then potassium is also low. Low levels of sodium and potassium relative to calcium and magnesium is seen in slow metabolic types and is an indicator of adrenal insufficiency. Adrenal insufficiency is commonly associated with conditions such as hypoglycemia, chronic fatigue, hypothyroidism, and viruses. Low blood pressure, fatigue and depression are also associated with adrenal insufficiency.

High tissue levels of of sodium and potassium relative to calcium and magnesium is indicative of high adrenal activity. This pattern is associated with an increase stress response and is common in fast metabolic types. Hyperthyroidism, hypertension, cardiovascular disease, and anxiety are other symptoms related to high tissue sodium and potassium.

The ratio of sodium to potassium is also important. Ideally, the TMA ratio should be 2.4:1. When sodium is high in relation to potassium, it may indicate an acute stress reaction or the beginning of an inflammatory process. When sodium is low relative to potassium, an exhaustion stage of stress may be ensuing. When sodium and potassium are out of balance with each other, either high or low, a kidney involvement may be present.

Conclusion

Routine determination of sodium and potassium in the blood cannot be relied upon for predicting sodium sensitive or sodium insensitive individuals unless a chronic or severe pathology is present. Individuals with high blood pressure will usually not show any deviation in these electrolytes in their blood. However, TMA may be used as a screening tool for assessing a pre-existing tendency for the development of high blood pressure related to sodium chloride sensitivity.

References

Kleiner, I.S., Orten, J.M. **Biochemistry**. C.V. Mosby, St Louis, 1962.

Brody, T. **Nutritional Biochemistry**. Academic Press, N.Y. 1994

Wilson, E.D., Fisher, K.. H., Garcia, P.A. **Principles of Nutrition** 4th. Ed. Wiley, N.Y., 1979.

Present Knowledge In Nutrition, 5th Ed. The Nutr. Found. Wash., D.C., 1984.

Fuller, C.M., Benos, D.J. The physiology and biochemistry of sodium and chloride permeability pathways in epithelia. **J. Nutr. Biochem**. 2, 1991.

Greger, J.L., Tseng, E. Longitudinal changes during the development of hypertension in rats fed excess chloride and sodium. **Soc. Exp. Biol. and Med**. 203, 1992.

Bergoff, R.S., Geraci, A.S. The influence of sodium chloride on blood pressure. **I.M.J.**, 56, 1929.

Morgan, T.D. The effect of potassium and bicarbonate ions on the rise in blood pressure caused by sodium chloride. **Clin. Sci.**, 63, 1982.

Shore, A.C., Markandu, N.D., MacGregor, G.A. Sodium loading in patients with essential hypertension. **Proc. Am. Soc. Hypert**. 2;78, 1987.

Kurtz, T.W., et al. "Salt-sensitive" essential hypertension in man: Is the sodium ion alone important? **N.E.J.M.**, 317, 1987.

Light, K., et al. Psychological strress induces sodium and fluid retention in men at high risk for hypertension.

'Quiz-show' tests link stress with hypertension; cut salt, fluid output. **Med. World News**, May 23, 1983.

Medeiros, D.M., Pellum, L.K. Elevation of cadmium, lead, and zinc in the hair of adult black female hypertensives. **Bul. Environ. Contam. Toxicol.**, 32, 1984.

Watts, D.L. The assessment of hypertensive tendencies from hair trace element analysis. **Chiro. Econ.**, 1989.

Altura, B.M., et al. Magnesium aspartate HCL (Mg -Asp) treatment ameliorates DOCA-salt hypertension.

Moore, T.J. The role of dietary electrolytes in hypertension. **J. Am Col. Nutr**. 8,5, 1989.

Patki, P.S., et al. Efficacy of potassium and magnesium in essential hypertension: A double blind. placebo controlled, crossover study. **Brit. Med. J**. 301, Sept., 1990.

Siani, A., et al. Controlled trial of long term oral potassium supplements in patients with mild hypertension. **Brit. Med. J**. 924, 1987.

Lasaridis, A.N., et al. Calcium diet supplementation increases urinary sodium excretion in essential hypertension. **Nephron** 45;250, 1987.
Dietary calcium in human hypertension. **Science,** 217, Jul., 1982.
Grobbee, D.E., Hofman, A. Effect of calcium supplementation on diastolic blood pressure in young people with mild hypertension. **Lancet,** Sept. 27, 1986.
Oparil, S., et al. Dietary Ca^{2+} prevents NaCl-sensitive hypertension in spontaneously hypertensive rats via sympatholytic and renal effects. **Am. J. Clin. Nutr.** 54, 1991.
Guyton, A.C. **Textbook of Medical Physiology.** Saunders, Phil., 1971.
Schullkin, J. **Sodium Hunger: the search for a salty taste.** Cambridge Univ. Press, N.Y. 1991.
Moore, R.D., Webb, G.D. **The K Factor.** Macmillan Pub., N.Y. 1986.

Chapter 14

Toxic And Other Metals

Toxic metals are minerals that do not have any known biological functions and are considered poisonous to biological system. They are often referred to as heavy metals due to their high atomic weights and they tend to displace the lighter nutritional metals, such as zinc, calcium, iron, etc.

Human hair has been accepted as an effective tissue for biological monitoring of toxic heavy metals by the U.S. Environmental Protection Agency and is being used for this purpose throughout the world. It is ideal because it fits the following criteria: 1) Hair accumulates all the important trace elements; 2) It is a commonly available tissue; 3) It is widespread geographically; 4) Hair is easily collected, stored and transported; 5) It is suitable since specimens can be resampled; 6) It is present in polluted and non-polluted areas; 7) The content of the hair correlates with environmental gradients of metals; and 8) There is sufficient background and exposure data. Hair is especially suitable for biological monitoring for exposure assessment as well as global, regional, and local surveillance monitoring and has advantages over other tissues. Monitoring metals in the urine measures the component that is not absorbed but excreted. The blood measures the component that is absorbed and temporarily in circulation before it is excreted and/or sequestered into storage depots.

Blood serum or urine testing can give an indication of the status of the body only at a specific time or over time if it is used on a daily basis. Trace element concentrations of the hair represent time-weighted exposure values that make it more useful for epidemiological and nutritional studies. Hair testing is also well suited for environmental and forensic investigations.

Lead (Pb)

Lead is probably the most notable toxic heavy metal and has been present throughout civilization. The ancient Egyptians used it in various forms, from a cooling plaster for skin conditions to cosmetics. The Roman Empire used lead to such an extent that it was once known as the Roman metal. Its soft and malleable characteristics made it ideal for use in forming pipes to carry water as well as eating and drinking utensils. Adding lead to wine was a common practice with the Romans. Artist paints were pigmented with lead. It has been speculated that the artist Van Gogh was poisoned by lead from extensive contact with his paints which may have contributed to the deterioration of his mental state. Unfortunately, lead has remained with us in more modern times.

Lead water pipes have been used extensively in our major cities and are still in use. Every year there are reports of lead contamination of drinking water in homes. The use of lead in the past as a gasoline anti-knock additive contributed greatly to the atmospheric pollution of lead. Lead has even been found in the polar ice caps, directly attributed to combustion of gasoline. Lead based interior house paints were extensively used throughout the U.S. Fortunately lead has been removed from gasoline and paints, but the dangers of lead toxicity from house paints remain. About one-third of the family dwellings in the United States were built before 1940, and over one-half of our present housing was built before 1960. Lead based paint may have been used in the majority of these homes since legislation limiting the use of lead based paint was not enacted until 1971. Many old or historic homes have several coats of lead based paints that are a source of lead toxicity in families who renovate these structures. Soils are also found high in lead as a result of automobile exhaust when lead was added to gasoline, particularly in densely populated cities. When vacated buildings in these areas are demolished leaded dust often settles in yards and playgrounds. This again is a source of lead contamination in children. Children are more susceptible to lead toxicity than adults as their body size cannot handle the same amount of exposure as an adult. In addition, they tend to retain more lead than adults due to their metabolic characteristic. Children are also short and are therefore closer to the ground where lead lingers. They may also inhale or ingest dust filled with lead from playgrounds.

Lead intake from pottery is also a source of toxicity. Recently a family was found to have excessive lead levels from storing orange juice in ceramic pottery. The acidic juice leached the lead from the container. Pottery that is of poor quality or cracked should not be used as food or beverage containers. Beverages stored in lead crystal containers are also a source of lead. Other sources include cosmetics, pesticides, metal polish, glass production, industry, smelters, battery manufacturing, and electroplating. Some hair dyes that blacken the hair contain lead acetate.

Early signs of lead exposure in adults may be vague and include symptoms such as fatigue, abdominal discomfort, vertigo, headaches, joint pains, poor coordination, and memory impairment. Chronic symptoms that can develop include anorexia, colic, muscle weakness and peripheral neuropathies (numbness and tingling in the extremities), long term memory deficits, psychomotor dysfunction, emotional instability, and hostility. Lead poisoning or "plumbism" can leave a dark gray line on the gums called a "lead line." Moderate levels of lead can contribute to immune suppression, kidney disorders, arthritis, hypertension, and stillbirths.

The effects of lead on the nervous system have implicated it as a major contributor to hyperactivity, learning disabilities, behavioral disorders, attention deficit, seizures and decreased IQ. Reports have implicated lead in the Sudden Infant Death Syndrome (SIDS). It was found that the incidence of SIDS followed increased air levels of lead by one or two months. Tissue studies of infants who died of SIDS revealed higher lead concentrations than those who died of other causes.

Lead displaces calcium and is deposited in bone through the ends or joints. Lead can destroy the normal cartilage tissue and contribute to arthritis. Since the teeth are similar to bone, lead exposure can increase the formation of dental caries in children. Dentists have related to me that children who develop cavities in large numbers are often hyperactive. It is possible that these children are toxic with lead.

Hair analysis is very helpful in screening for lead contamination. In many cases it is more useful than blood analysis. When lead is ingested, the body will attempt to remove it immediately. If the body is unable to eliminate the metal, then it will be sequestered into storage tissues, such as the liver, kidney, and bone. Lead can deposit virtually anywhere within the body but has a particular affinity for bone. If ongoing exposure is not occurring, then the majority of lead will eventually be cleared from the blood. After that time, a person with an accumulation of lead in tissue may not show significant lead levels in the blood. However, lead deposited in the tissues will show in the hair.

When evaluating lead in the hair, we are concerned not only with the level, but also its relationship or ratio with other elements. We have established the TMA calcium to lead ratio at a minimum of 84:1. Iron is also antagonistic to lead. The Fe/Pb ratio should be a minimum of 4.4:1. When a reduction is found in these ratios, lead is considered a potential health hazard.

Arsenic (As)

Arsenic has a long history with man. It was once used as a medication for treating various aliments. Napoleon was suspected to be poisoned by arsenic, which was commonly used during this time to remove one's enemies. This is controversial however. His physical and mental symptoms could have been related to arsenic poisoning, and his hair sample did show a high arsenic level. However, investigators found that the wallpaper in his home contained very high amounts of arsenic that could have been the source of his exposure rather than from covert poisoning.

Arsenic has been found in seafoods obtained from coastal waters, particularly shrimp, oysters, and mussels. Other sources include arsenic rich soils, arsenic containing insect sprays, and burning of arsenate treated building materials in fireplaces. Coal combustion and smelters are other common sources of arsenic. Arsenic has been found in opium samples and consequently high in the hair of opium addicts.

Symptoms of acute arsenic toxicity include:
- Nausea
- Diarrhea
- Burning sensation of mouth and throat
- Vomiting
- Abdominal pain

Symptoms of chronic arsenic toxicity include:
- Dermatitis
- Respiratory tract irritation
- Muscle aches
- Headaches
- Weakness
- Convulsions
- Hyperpigmentation of the skin
- Neuropathy
- Anemia
- Pigmentation of nails
- Drowsiness
- Confusion
- Increases risk of skin, lung, and liver cancers

Arsenic antagonizes sulfur and selenium and may contribute to a deficiency of these minerals as well as increase the requirements for vitamin E.

Beryllium (Be)

Beryllium is considered a toxin usually from coal burning industry or manufacturing. High levels have been associated with rickets and therefore may interfere with calcium and other calcium related minerals as well as vitamin D. Beryllium is associated with pneumonitis and increased incidence of lung cancer in exposed workers. Excess accumulation adversely affects cell division, synthesis of DNA, enzyme activation and gene expression.

Cadmium (Cd)

Cadmium is given off by the burning of petrochemicals, plastics, and tires. Smelters, cadmium plating and battery manufacturing are sources of cadmium as well as tobacco. It is used as a stabilizer for PVC pipes and as a pigment in paints. The concentration in soils has been rising due to the increased atmospheric levels and the use of cadmium containing fertilizer. This of course increases the cadmium content of the foods grown in these soils.

Cadmium is a neurotoxin and adversely affects a number of enzymes. Conditions associated with cadmium toxicity include bone and kidney disease, hypercholesterol, hypertension, emphysema, headaches, and reproductive disorders. Cadmium deposits on the surface of bones can cause pain in the middle of the bones rather than in the joints. Exposure or removal of cadmium from the body can produce flu-like symptoms.

The major antagonist to cadmium is zinc. The ideal TMA ratio of zinc to cadmium should be a minimum of 500:1.

Mercury (Hg)

Like arsenic, mercury has been used medicinally. Doctors who dispensed the silvery medicine were known as quacks. This was a term that developed due to the shortening of the name quicksilver. Mercury was found in calomel lotion and was the basis for mercurial diuretics. The most well recognized condition associated with mercury toxicity is "hatters shakes." Years ago individuals working in hat factories were exposed to mercury during the processing of felt. A well-known character of Alice In Wonderland was apparently one of these workers, the "Mad Hatter."

Mercury has been found in skin lightening creams. Individuals have developed kidney disturbances due to the absorption of the mercury through the skin. Contaminated fish are also a source of mercury. Accumulation from these sources show up readily in the hair. Mercury amalgams contain mercury and may also contribute to exposure. It is used as a constituent of fungicides, algaecides, and insecticides. These have contributed to mercury contamination of foods, particularly grains and cereals. Paper products and lumber contain mercury to inhibit fungus. Families have been reported to develop symptoms of mercury toxicity during the winter months from burning newspaper and building materials in their fireplaces. The mercury vapor was given off during combustion.

Mercury accumulates in tissues such as the kidneys, eyes, brain, thyroid, and liver. It is not uncommon to find people with hypothyroidism to have mercury toxicity. Excess mercury has been implicated in the formation of cataracts. Other symptoms of mercury toxicity include:

Weakness of the hands	Irritability
Headaches (band type)	Rashes
Paraesthesis	Speech difficulties
Retinitis	Joint pain
Blushing	Excess salivation

Cerebral palsy and mental retardation have been associated with mercury toxicity in children.

Nutritional modification can help protect from the adverse effects of heavy metals. Zinc, selenium, iron, and sulfur are particularly helpful in combatting and preventing the adverse effects of mercury. The TMA zinc to mercury ratio should be at least 200:1, iron to mercury 22:1, selenium to mercury 0.8:1, and sulfur to mercury 28000:1. Proteins and sulfur-containing amino acids are helpful in combating mercury. Garlic is especially high in sulfur-containing amino acids.

Aluminum (Al)

Excess aluminum can contribute to a deterioration of mental function. Termed dialysis dementia, the condition has been found in individuals receiving dialysis treatment from which they accumulate high amounts of aluminum. Excess aluminum has also been implicated in the development of Alzheimer's disease. Aluminum can adversely affect mental function and bone integrity, as well as inhibit important enzyme systems in the body and interfere with normal immune function.

The absorption of aluminum can be enhanced in the presence of increased para-thyroid activity. This usually accompanies low thyroid activity and imbalances in normal nutritional status.

A major source of aluminum has been through the use of aluminum cooking utensils, aluminum foil, and baking powder. Antacids have been a contributor as well as antiperspirants and contaminated water supplies. Aluminum is often used as a buffering agent in medications and may be found in herbs.

ULTRA TRACE ELEMENTS

Antimony (Sb)

There is presently no clinical significance of low TMA antimony levels and toxicity symptoms have not yet been recognized. However, high TMA levels may indicate unnecessary exposure that may be investigated further. The most common sources are from industry and metallurgy.

Barium (Ba)

Barium has not been shown to be an essential mineral. High levels of barium in water supplies have been associated with high blood pressure and cardiovascular disease. Biological significance of low TMA levels cannot be described at this time.

Boron (B)

Boron is thought to be related to endocrine activity, especially those that affect calcium metabolism. Boron is also thought to have an estrogenic effect. However, studies of post menopausal women on a low boron diet that were supplemented with over three milligrams per day of boron revealed no change in minerals or steroid levels. Animal studies suggest that boron is more synergistic to vitamin D. Deficiency of this element in humans has not been identified. Significance of low TMA levels is unknown at this time. Signs of acute boron toxicity in humans include:

Nausea	Vomiting
Diarrhea	Dermatitis
Lethargy	

Excess boron antagonizes vitamin B_2 and contributes to urinary losses of the vitamin. Fruits, vegetables, legumes and tubers are high in boron. Water may also be high in boron and varies considerably across the country. Other sources are found in analgesics, antibiotics, decongestants, antihistamines, laxatives, antacids and insecticide dust.

Cobalt (Co)

A deficiency of cobalt can result from low intake, poor absorption and high iron intake. Increased bacterial colonization of the small intestine is known to inhibit cobalt absorption as well as enteritis, and achlorhydria (lack of Intrinsic Factor). Parasites, particularly fish tape worms, selectively inhibit cobalt absorption. Medications may interfere with cobalt absorption such as colchicine, and neomycin. Symptoms of cobalt deficiency other than anemia include:

Demylination	Dorsal and lateral columns atrophy
Paresthesia of extremities	Personality and mood swings
Loss of joint-position sense	Decreased vibratory sense
Sore tongue	Diarrhea
Numbness in heels radiating to legs	Numbness in fingertips radiating into arms
Abnormalities in cutaneous touch, pain, reflexes, and gait	Sharp pain in feet when head is flexed anteriorly (Lhermitte's Sign)

Some enzymes may be affected by cobalt deficiency such as alkaline phosphatase. Urinary methylmalonic acid and homocysteine may be increased due to a lack of cobalt activated enzymes L-methylmalonyl-CoA mutase and methionine senthetase.

Hyperthyroidism apparently increases the requirement for this trace element. Cobalt is known to reduce thyroid activity and may prove beneficial in hyperthyroid conditions. Cobalt has been reported to lower blood pressure in hypertensive patients.

Patients with neurological disease such as Parkinson's, multiple sclerosis and neuropsychiatric conditions have been reported to respond well to cobalt therapy. The response to supplementation was noted even though the patients showed no clinical signs of cobalt deficiency such as anemia. This indicates the effects of a subclinical cobalt deficiency.

Excess cobalt has been associated with anemia due to a cobalt/iron antagonism. Observed symptoms of cobalt toxicity include:

Flushing	Deafness
Chest Pains	Polycythemia
Dermatitis	Hyperglycemia
Nausea	Hypothyroidism
Vomiting	Cardiac (Congestive Failure)
Kidney problems	Thyroid hyperplasia
Thyroid disturbance	

Acute Symptoms:

Gastrointestinal disturbances	Abdominal pain
Vomiting	

Other than through supplements, excess cobalt may develop in areas of high cobalt soils and water. Industrial exposures to cobalt have occurred in workers involved in grinding or sharpening operations. Cobalt is added to alloys to produce extremely hard metals. Other exposures have been identified with diamond polishing, production of paint pigments, drying agents in paint, enameling and electroplating. Symptoms of excessive exposure in workers have been described and include asthma and lung disease. The richest food source of this element is found in green leafy vegetables.

Germanium (Ge)

Little is known concerning the biological functions of germanium. Clinical significance cannot be placed on low TMA levels at this time.

Excessive intake of germanium has been reported to adversely affect kidney function.

Gold (Au)

Gold has no known function in biological systems. Symptoms of gold toxicity have been described in patients receiving gold compounds for the treatment of pain associated with arthritis.

Dermatitis	Stomatitis
Anemia	Renal Dysfunction
Aplastic Anemia	Hematuria
Albuminuria	Thrombocytopenia
Eosinophilia	Gastrointestinal Discomfort

Lithium (Li)

Lithium is felt to have some role in human metabolism but requires more research. Significance of low TMA lithium levels has yet to be determined.

Excess lithium may be associated with therapeutic lithium treatment. Lithium supplementation is used for treating emotional disorders, particularly manic depression. Lithium is also found naturally occurring in water supplies. Too much lithium can interfere with iodine uptake by the thyroid gland, and may block thyroxin release or thyroid stimulating hormone (TSH). Lithium is known to alter the intra-to extra-cellular potassium ratio. This may result in a loss of intracellular potassium and contribute to hyperkalemia. Other conditions associated with chronic lithium excess include: renal induced diabetes insipidus, hair loss, hypercalcuria, inability to acidify the urine, leukocytosis, and eosinophilia. Chronic lithium accumulation has been associated with the following conditions:

Diabetes insipidus	Osteoporosis
Hair loss	Leukocytosis
Eosinophilia	Hyperkalemia
Hypothyroidism	Fatigue
Weight gain	Goiter

Hypothyroidism is a well known side effect of excess lithium. The thyroid is inhibited by the lithium induced hyper parathyroid activity. Chronic lithium excess can therefore result in elevated serum calcium and reduced serum phosphorus.

Molybdenum (Mo)

Although this mineral is known to activate some enzymes and is involved in purine metabolism and iron utilization, very little is known about molybdenum deficiency in humans. A deficiency is known to increase the incidence of dental caries. This metal has been shown to be beneficial in the treatment of dental problems caused by fluorosis and is considered to be mutually antagonistic to fluoride.

Molybdenum inhibits calcium transport into bones. Excesses also reduce the normal elasticity of connective tissues such as tendons and can contribute to joint stiffness. Other symptoms associated with molybdenum excess include gout, arthralgia, and increased uric acid levels. Excess molybdenum antagonizes copper and sulfur, particularly methionine and cystine. Reduced glucose-6-phosphate and increased xanthine oxidase activity is seen with molybdenum excess. Molybdenum is found in all foods but the highest sources are found in milk, legumes, and cereals.

Sources of molybdenum other than supplements include:

Water	Mining
Milling	Lubricants
Paints	Fertilizers
Stainless steel	Armor plating

The molybdenum-copper antagonism may contribute to copper deficiency conditions that include:

Hypercholesterolemia	Gout
Hypoparathyroidism	Hypertension
Low Estrogen/Progesterone ratio.	

Enhanced adrenal and thyroid activity can increase the excretion of copper thereby allowing excessive accumulation of molybdenum, even without a high dietary intake of molybdenum.

Nickel (Ni)

Nickel is found in most biological systems. The metal has an influence on carbohydrate metabolism, is associated with some enzyme activity, and is thought to stabilize the protein structure of these enzymes. Nickel has been found to cause hypoglycemia by prolonging the action of insulin. More is known about nickel's toxic effects than deficiency, although it has been established by animal studies to be an essential element.

Years ago poisoning of workers in a nickel factory resulted in increased lung cancer as a result of breathing a form of nickel dust. Nickel antagonizes the effects of adrenaline and other adrenal hormones and acts as an antidiuretic. Observations of TMA studies indicate that nickel increases the retention of sodium and in conjunction with its antidiuretic effects can promote water retention. One of the most common and well-known effects of nickel toxicity is contact dermatitis. Nickel is associated with and produces more instances of allergic dermatitis than any other metal. We typically find individuals who have contact dermatitis to metals have had their ears pierced. Following ear piercing, a cheap grade of a metal post is usually inserted into the opening. When the puncture site becomes infected, there is apparently an increased absorption of nickel from the metal. Afterwards, contact dermatitis may develop to any metal containing nickel. These include wrist watches, necklaces, zippers, eyeglass rims, coins, safety pins and even metal shoe eyelets. For some women the only way to avoid this reaction is to wear gold jewelry of at least 14 karat. The better the gold quality, the less nickel is present. It should be noted that most women do not mind this inconvenience.

Other sources of nickel are cooking utensils, metal implants, water run through nickel plated faucets, electroplating, glass paint, alkaline batteries, insecticides, fuel additives, ceramics, electrical wiring, and pigments in paints and wallpaper. Nickel is also used in the dying of printed fabrics, which when washed can be liberated by detergents.

Food may also be a source of nickel. Nickel is used as a catalyst in the hydrogenation process that solidifies fats, such as shortening and margarine. Foods highest in nickel include whole grains, cocoa, legumes, oysters, and margarine. Tea is very high in nickel. High TMA nickel is often seen in individuals who consume large amounts of teas. Ingestion of these foods has been reported to produce skin eruptions in nickel sensitive individuals.

Platinum (Pt)

There are no known biological requirements for platinum. Toxic signs of platinum have not been described. However, high levels may indicate excessive and unnecessary exposure. Sources are largely from mining, catalytic converters and jewelry making. Platinum is a constituent of some dental alloys, and has been found elevated in patients taking platinum containing anti-tumor drugs such as cisplatin. Treatment with the platinum containing drug increased the excretion of magnesium.

Silicon (Si)

A deficiency of silicon has not been identified in man. However, animal studies have shown that this mineral appears to play a role in maintenance of connective tissues and bone calcification during the development stage. Experimental studies have revealed that silicon is decreased in the arterial walls with atherosclerosis. The level of silicon also decreases in the skin with age. Silicon is synergistic to copper in connective tissue formation and integrity. High fiber grains, cereals, and fruits are good sources of silicon. Beer may also contain significant amounts of this element.

Silicosis has been described in miners. Inhaled silicon produces lesions in the lungs similar to the effects of asbestos. Excess silicon has also been related to renal stone formation. Silicon has been implicated in collagen disorders and immunological disturbances in women having leaky breast implants.

Strontium (Sr)

Strontium has not been found to be necessary for normal biological functions and is not considered an essential element.

Strontium is apparently antagonistic to calcium and can therefore interfere with normal calcium metabolism. Observations of TMA patterns have shown high levels of strontium in females with a history of malignancy.

Sulfur (S)

The majority of sulfur in the diet is obtained from protein, particularly the sulfur containing amino acids, cystine, cysteine, and methionine foods, such as fish, meats, chicken, etc. Low levels may indicate low protein in the diet or poor digestion and absorption of proteins.

Sulfur is known to reduce the effects of selenium toxicity as well as antagonize heavy metals. Low sulfur to heavy metal ratios may indicate an increased requirement for sulfur protein, such as low sulfur/lead, sulfur/mercury, sulfur/cadmium, and sulfur/copper.

Silver (Ag)

Low levels of silver are insignificant since there appears to be no requirement for this trace element in biological systems.

Silver is found with mining of ores, some industry, x-ray films, as well as jewelry and flatware. Silver is known to antagonize selenium and vitamin E in animals. Excess levels may contribute to free radical production and increase the requirement for these nutrients.

Silver is known to possess anti-bacterial properties and is often impregnated in charcoal water filters, as well as being taken in a colloidal form. Its use for these purposes may produce elevated hair levels of the mineral.

Tin (Sn)

Significance of low TMA tin cannot be ascertained at this time. Although, tin in excess interferes with iron metabolism and produces heme breakdown. It also increases the excretion of selenium and zinc.

Titanium (Ti)

Presently there is no indication of titanium being necessary in biological functions. Significance cannot be placed upon a low TMA level at this time.

There are no known toxicity indications for titanium. Titanium is used in alloys related to dental and other metal prosthetic devices.

Vanadium (V)

There are no known effects of vanadium deficiency. Excess vanadium is known to inhibit cholesterol formation as well as some amino acids, or proteins. Decreased hormone production and selective protein deficiency could occur with excessive accumulation of this element. Vanadium antagonizes the mineral chromium and could lead to blood sugar disturbances. In animal studies vanadium has been demonstrated to reduce coenzyme A and coenzyme Q levels, as well as uncouple oxidative phosphorylation, and raise monoamine oxidase (MAO) activity. These effects were nullified by chromium.

Vanadium is antagonistic to sulfur amino acids. In human studies, excess vanadium intake inhibited cholesterol synthesis by way of squalene synthetase enzyme inhibition. However, vanadium had no beneficial effect in lowering lipid levels in patients suffering from hypercholesterolemia or ischemic heart disease. Vanadium is also an antagonistic to vitamin C and hemoglobin synthesis. Sources of Vanadium include:

- Petroleum refining
- Boiler cleaning
- Soil
- Metal refining
- Water

Vanadium toxicity produces symptoms similar to respiratory tract infections. Acute toxicity can produce a greenish discoloration of the tongue. A group of villagers in Thailand were found to have health conditions associated with excess vanadium due to high levels in the soil and water. Symptoms included kidney stones, periodic paralysis due to low blood potassium, diabetes and death. Vanadium is also suspected to be a neurotoxin through increased free radical production and lipid peroxidation.

Zirconium (Zr)

Zirconium has not been recognized as an essential element, and toxicity of zirconium has not been described in humans. Zirconium has been determined to be biocompatible and may be used in metal implants.

References

Jenkins, D.W. Biological monitoring of toxic trace metals Vol. 1. Biological monitoring and surveillance. **EPA** 600/3-80-089, 1980
Clin. Chem. 36,3, 1990
Niculescu, T., et al. Relationship between the lead concentration in hair and occupational exposure. **Brit. J. Industrial Med.** 40, 67, 1983.
Medeiros, D.M., Pellum, L.K. Elevation of cadmium, lead, and zinc in the hair of adult black female hypertensives. **Bull. Environ. Toxicol.** 32, 1984.
Clarke, A.N., Wilson, D.J. Preparation of hair for lead analysis. **Arch. Environ. Hlth.** 28, 1974.
Cheraskin, E., Ringsdorf, W.M. The distribution of lead in human hair. **J. of Med. Assoc. of Alabama.** April, 1979.
Cheraskin, E., Ringsdorf, W.M. Prevalence of possible lead toxicity as determined by hair analysis. **J. Orthomol. Psych.** 8,2
Baaumslag, N., et al. Trace metal content of maternal and neonate hair. Zinc, copper, iron, and lead. **Arch. Environ. Hlth.** 29, 1974.
Watts, D.L. Prevalence of lead in environment threatens children. **Hlth. Freedom** News. Oct. 1985.
Watts, D.L. Implications of lead toxicity. **TEI Newsletter.** 1,2, 1985.
Grazino, J.H., Blum, C. Lead exposure from lead crystal. **Lancet.** 337, 1991.
Sharp, D.S., Smith, A.H. Elevated blood pressure in treated hypertensives with low-level lead accumulation. **Arch. Environ. Hlth.** 44,1, 1989.
Batuman, V., et al. Contribution of lead to hypertension with renal impairment. **N.E.J.M.** 309, 1, 1983.
Annest, J.I., et al. Chronological trend in blood lead levels between 1976 and 1980. **N.E.J.M.** 308, 23, 1983.
Florence, T.M., Lilley, S.G., Stauber, J.L. Skin absorption of lead. **Lancet.** Jul. 16, 1988.
Baker, E.L., et al. A nationwide survey of heavy metal absorption in children living near primary copper, lead and zinc smelter. **Am. J. Epidemiology.** 206, 4, 1977.
Jones, R.J. The continuing hazard of lead in drinking water. **Lancet** Sept. 16, 1989.
Kopito, L., et al. Chronic plumbism in children. Diagnosed by hair analysis. **J.A.M.A** 209,2, 1969.

Nriagu, J.O. **Lead and Lead Poisoning in Antiquity**. Wiley, N.Y., 1983.

Matte, T.D., et al. Acute high-dose lead exposure from beverage contaminated by traditional Mexican pottery. **Lancet** 344, 8929, 1994.

Alexander. The uptake of lead by children in differing environments. **Environ. Hlth. Prospectus.** 1974.

Lead absorption my provide clue to Sudden Infant Death Syndrome. **Med. World News.** Oct., 1983.

Erickson, et al. Tissue mineral levels in victims of Sudden Infant Death Syndrome 1. Toxic metals - lead and cadmium. **Ped. Res.** 17, 10, 1983.

Cheraskin, E., Ringsdorf, M. Prevalence of possible lead toxicity as determined by hair analysis. **J. Orthomol. Psych.** 8, 2.

Am. J. Ind. Med. 2,1, 5-14, 1981.

Westhoff, D.D., et al. Arsenic Intoxication As a Cause of Megaloblastic Anemia. **Blood** 75,45, 2. 241-246

Narang, A.P.S., et al. Arsenic levels in opium eaters in India. **Trace Elements in Med.** 4,4, 1987.

Peters, HA, et al. Seasonal Arsenic Exposure From Burning Treated Wood. **J.A.M.A.** 11;25,18, 2393-2396, 1984.

Aller, A.J. The clinical significance of beryllium. **J. Trace Elements and Electrolytes in Health and Dis.** 4,1, 1990.

Ashby, J., et al. Studies on the genotoxicity of beryllium sulphate in vitro and in vivo. **Mutation Res.** 240, 3, 1990.

Walker, P.R., LeBlanc, J., Sikorska, M. Effects of aluminum and other cations on the structure of brain and liver chromatin. **Biochem.** 28,9, 1989.

Marlowe, M., Mood, C. Hair aluminum concentration and nonadaptive classroom behavior. **J. of Advancement in Med.** 1,3, 1988.

Yokel, R.A. Hair as an indicator of excessive aluminum exposure. Clin. Chem. 28, 4, 1982.

Altmann, P., et al. Disturbance of cerebral function by aluminum in haemodialysis patients without overt aluminum toxicity. **Lancet.** Jul, 1989.

Birchall. J.D., Chappell, J.S. Aluminum, chemical physiology and Alzheimer's disease. **Lancet.** Oct, 1988.

Pearl, D.P., et al. Intraneuronal aluminum accumulation in Amyotrophic Lateral Sclerosis and Parkinsonism-Dementia of Guam. **Science.** 217, 1982.

Boyce, B.F. et al. Hypercalcaemic osteomalacia due to aluminum toxicity. **Lancet.** Nov, 1982.

Garrett, P.J., et al. Aluminum encephalopathy: Clinical and immunological features. **Quart. J. Med.** 69, 258, 1988.

Beattie, J.H., Peace, H.S. The influence of a low-boron diet and boron supplementation on bone, major mineral and sex steroid metabolism in postmenopausal women. **Brit. J. Nutr.** 69,3, 1993

King, N., et al. The effect of in ovo boron supplementation on bone mineralization of the vitamin D-deficient chicken embryo. **Biol. Trace Element Res.** 31,1, 1991.

Hunt, C.D., Shuler, T.R., Mullen, L.M. Concentration of boron and other elements in human foods and personal-care products. **J. Am. Diet. Assoc.** 91,5, 1991.

Trace Elements In Human And Animal Nutrition 5th Ed. Mertz, W. Academic Press, NY, 1986.

Tracey, J.P., Schiffman, F.J. Magnetic resonance imaging in cobalamin deficiency. **Lancet.** 339. 1992.

Cobalamin Biochemistry and Pathophysiology. Babior, B.M., Ed. John Wiley Pub. N.Y., 1975.

Domingo, J.L. Cobalt in the environment and its toxicological implications. **Reviews of Environmental Contamination and Toxicology.** 108, 1989.

Lindenbaum, J., et al. Neuropsychiatric disorders caused by cobalamin deficiency in the absence of anemia or macrocytosis. **N.E.J.M.** Jun. 30, 1988.

Disorders Of Mineral Metabolism Vol. I. Bronner, Coburn, Eds. Academic Press, NY, 1981.

Trace Elements In Human Health And Disease Vol II. Prasad, AS, Ed. Academic Press, N.Y., 1976.

Trace Elements In Human and Animal Nutrition. Underwood, E.J. Academic Press, NY., 1977.

Teodorescu, V., et al. Gold -induced colitis: a case report and review of the literature. **Mt. Sinai J. of Med.** 60,3, 1993.

Perrild, H., et al. Thyroid function and ultrasonically determined thyroid size in patients receiving long-term lithium treatment. **Am. J. Psychiatry,** 147, 1 1990.

Chen, Y., Silverstone, T. Lithium and weight gain. **Int. Clin. Psychopharmacology,** 5,3, 1990.

Yao, Z.M., Zhang, L.H. Microelement-molybdenum and its use for the treatment of children's fluorine-stained teeth. **Chinese J. of Preventive Med.** 26, 1, 1992.

An essential role for nickel. **Med. World News.** Apr., 1972.

Fisher, A.A. Nickel dermatitis. Dermatology. Dec. 1981.
Sunderman, F.W. Nickel. **Disorders of Mineral Metabolism Vol. I.** Bronner, F., Coburn, J.W., Eds. Academic Press, N.Y., 1981.
Kanematsu, N., et al. Mutagenicity of cadmium, platinum and rhodium compounds in cultured mammalian cells. **Gifu Shika Zasshi** 17,2, 1990.
Minami, T., et al. Accumulation of platinum in the intervertebral discs and vertebrae of ovarian tumor-bearing patinets treated with cisplatin. **Biol. Trace Element Res.** 42, 1994.
Zumkley, H.P., et al. Influence of cisplatin on renal function and zinc, copper, and magnesium excretion. **Trace Substances in Environmental Health XVI.** Hemphill, D.D., Ed. Univ. Mo. 1992.
Emerick, R.J., Kayongo-Male, H. Silicon facilitation of copper utilization in the rat. **J. Nutr. Biochem.** 1, 1990.
Bignall, J. Silicone breast implants. breast feeding and scleroderma. **Lancet.** 343, Jan. 1994.
Bellia, J.P., Birchall. J.D., Roberts, N.B. Beer: a dietary source of silicon. **Lancet.** 343, Jan. 1994.
Silicon implants and autoimmune disease. **Lancet.** 343, Feb. 1994.
Breme, J., Wadewitz, V. Comparison of titanium-tantalum and titanium-niobium alloys for application as dental implants. **Int. J. Oral and Maxillofacial Implants**, 4,2, 1989.
Sitprija, V., et al. Metabolic problems in northeastern Thailand: possible role of vanadium. **Mineral and Electrolyte Metabol.** 19,1, 1993.
Sasi, M.M., et al. Microchromatographic analysis of lipids, protein, and occurrence of lipid peroxidation in various brain areas of vanadium exposed rats: a possible mechanism of vanadium neurotoxicity. **Neurotoxicology**, 14, 1, 1993.
Ghosh, S., Sharma, A., Talukder, G. Zirconium. An abnormal trace element in biology. **Biol. Trace Element Res.** 35,3, 1992.
Fujita, M. In vitro study on biocompatibility of zirconium and titanium. **J. of the Stomatological Soc.** Japan. 60,1, 1993.
Arch. Ind. Hyg. **Occupational Med.** 8, 1953.

Index

A

"absolute" deficiency 71
absolute zinc deficiency 100
absorption 16
achlorhydria 163
acid-alkali balance 147
acidosis 150
acrodermatitis enteropathica 4, 97
acute selenium toxicity symptoms in animals 133
Addison's disease 26, 62, 150
adrenal 39, 56, 112
adrenal activity 58
adrenal cortex 31, 73, 148
adrenal cortex (anabolic) 26
adrenal cortex (catabolic) 26
adrenal corticotrophic hormone (ACTH) 149
adrenal glands 35, 37, 53, 71
adrenal hormones 118
adrenal hyperactivity 54
adrenal insufficiency 54, 61, 153
adrenal medulla 26
adrenal status 153
adrenals 36, 60
adrenapause 54
adult onset diabetes 57, 60
advantages of hair TMA 8
aggressive behavior 107
aging 135
AIDS 42, 100, 136
alarm reaction 28
alarm stage of stress 28, 29
alcohol 66, 71, 100, 111, 119
alcoholic cirrhosis 71, 143
alcoholism 54
aldosterone 148
algaecides 161
alkali disease 132
alkaline phosphatase 10
allergic dermatitis 167
allergies 58, 83
allergies (histamine) 42
allergies (low histamine) 42
ALS 42, 111
aluminum (Al) 162
aluminum hydroxide 53
Alzheimer's disease 162
amphetamines 50
amylophagia 108
analgesics 163
anemia 15, 79, 107
aneurysms 82
angiotensin 148
anorexia 42
anorexia nervosa 84, 98
antacids 50, 53, 114, 162, 163
antagonistic relationship 15
anterior pituitary 26
anti-bacterial agents 50
anti-convulsants 50
anti-dandruff 7
anti-viral 87
antibiotic sensitivity 83
antibiotics 163
antibody formation 136
antidiuretic hormone (ADH) 149
antihistamines 163
antimony (Sb) 162
anxiety 42, 58, 59, 67, 153
anxious 67
apathy 67
apple-shaped 33, 36
apricots 45
arrhythmia 70
arsenic 159
arteriosclerosis 70
arthralgia 166
arthritis 30, 36, 69, 78, 79, 143, 158
arthritis (osteo type) 42
arthritis (rheumatoid) 42
assessment of selenium status 142
asthma 42
athero- and arteriosclerosis 68
atherosclerosis 70, 82, 125, 143
attention deficit 158
attention span 107
autism 100

B

bacterial infection 22, 28, 79, 80, 81, 86, 93, 104, 109
bamboo shoots 46
barium (Ba) 163
beet greens 45, 53
behavioral disorders 158
beryllium (Be) 160
beta blocking drug 49
biceps 62
biochemical individuality 33
bleaching of the hair 7
bleeding gums 93
blind staggers 132
blood glucose 124
blood pressure 42
blood sugar disorders 70
blood transfusions 110
body odor 67
body types 33, 41
bone 80
bone cortex 55
bone matrix 62
bone resorption 55
boron (B) 163
bowel resection 71
broccoli 46
bruising 93
brussel sprouts 46
bulemia 84

Index

"burn-out" 30
bursitis 69

C

cabbage 46
cadmium 2, 3, 10, 73, 80, 97, 150, 152, 160
caffeine 46, 47
calcification of cartilage 62
calcitonin 53
calcium 7, 10, 15, 16, 20, 21, 22, 26, 27, 37, 42, 43, 45, 50, 52, 53, 54, 55, 56, 57, 58, 59, 60, 61, 62, 67, 68, 73, 74, 86, 91, 102, 112, 152, 160
calcium accumulation 67
calcium blockers 67
calcium to lead ratio 159
cancer 34, 135
cancers 143
candida 38, 100
candidiasis 87
carbohydrate metabolism 124
carbohydrates 45
cardiovascular disease 4, 36, 43, 100, 125, 153
cardiovascular disorders 82
cassava 45
cataracts 134, 161
cauliflower 46
celiac disease 71
cellular oxidation 133
cellular respiration 82
cereals 45, 53, 58, 71
cerebral palsy 161
chard 45, 53
cheese 45
cherries 45
chickweed 111
children 47
chloride 147, 151
chloride-sensitive 151
chlorosis 107
chocolate 45
cholesterol 82, 86, 100
cholesterol synthesis 119
chromium 75, 124
chromium deficiency-diabetes 124
chromium requirements 129
chronic fatigue 153
chronic fatigue syndrome (CFS) 38, 60, 70, 86
chronic selenium toxicity symptoms in animals 133
cirrhosis 4, 110, 111
cisplatin 168
cobalt 114, 163
coenzyme A 170
coenzyme Q 170
coffee 46
cognitive functions 107
cola drinks 47
colchicine 163
colitis 30
collagen 62
collagen disorders 169
colon cancer 53
coma 150

comfrey 49
comfrey root 111
conditions associated with magnesium deficiency 70
confusion 150
congestive heart failure 70
conjunctivitis 62
constipation 62, 69, 84, 99
contact dermatitis 167
contamination of the hair 6
convulsions 70
copper 2, 4, 10, 15, 16, 20, 22, 39, 55, 56, 62, 81, 82, 84, 85, 86, 87, 97, 103, 111, 166
copper and anemia 79
copper and arthritis 79
copper and mental function 88
copper and the adrenal glands 91
copper and the thyroid 90
copper bracelets 78, 80
copper intrauterine devices 84
copper toxicity 83, 90
copper water pipes 83
corticosteroids 50
cortisone 53, 100
Crohn's Disease 136
Cushings disease 26, 54
cyanogenic glucosides 45
cystic fibrosis 4, 136
cystine 166
cytochrome c oxidase 78
cytomegleo virus 38, 60, 86

D

dairy foods 45
dairy products 54, 114
decongestants 163
dehydration 149
deltoids 62
dental abscess 81
dental caries 158
depression 28, 38, 59, 60, 62, 67, 84, 86, 99, 100
dermatitis 119
diabetes 4, 34, 36, 54, 57, 70, 98, 109, 124
diabetes (adult onset) 42
diabetes (juvenile) 42
diabetes insipidus 166
diabetic acidosis 71
diabetic neuropathy 143
dialysis dementia 162
diastolic high blood pressure 68
diet 24
digitalis 150
diuril 90
DNA 67, 107
dopamine 81
dopamine B-hydroxylase 78
Down's syndrome 117
drugs 135
dry skin 57
dwarfism 4
dyslexia 88
dysphagia 108

E

EBV 60
eclampsia 70, 85, 100
electrolytes 147
emotional volatility 84
emphysema 160
endocrine disorders 62
endocrine effects upon copper 90
endocrine glands 25
enteritis 163
environmental contamination 7
eosinophilia 166
ephedrine 50
epilepsy 117
epinephrine 50, 149
Epstein Barr virus 38, 60, 86
estrogen 25, 53, 55, 84, 85, 86, 90, 98, 99, 118, 126, 149
estrogenic effect 163
excessive perspiration 67
exhaustion 59
exhaustion stage of stress 30, 153
exudative diathesis 134

F

fast metabolic rate 42, 58
fast metabolic type 34, 43, 45, 151, 153
fast metabolizer 35, 36, 37, 38, 60
fatigue 38, 59, 60, 61, 62, 84, 86, 99
fats 45
Fe/Pb ratio 159
"fight or flight" 27, 28
fingernails 97
fluorosis 166
folic acid 75
food cravings 84
free radical formation 134
frontal headaches 84, 99
fungicides 161
fungus 38, 42, 87, 100

G

gallbladder obstruction 79
gallstones 57, 62, 69, 80, 85, 86
gasoline anti-knock additive 157
gastric ulcers 100
gastritis 30
geophagia 108
germanium 165
ginseng 49
Glanzmann's disease 135
glucose 124
glucose control 126
glucose-6-phosphate 166
glutathione peroxidase 133
gluteus medius 62
glycyrrhizic acid 48
goitrogens 45
gold 165
gout 83, 166
grains 45, 53, 58, 71, 100

growth hormones 4

H

hair analysis 3
hair dye 6
hair loss 166
hair sample 5
hamstrings 62
hard water 43
HDL 82, 100, 125
headaches 59, 108, 150, 160
hearing difficulties 62
heart arrhythmia 150
heart attack 126
heart disease 34, 68
heart enlargement 82
heart failure 82
heavy metals 2, 3, 135
hemochromatosis 110
hemoglobin 16
hemolytic anemia 135
hemolytic conditions 110
hemosiderosis 110
hepatitis 83, 122
herbs 48, 111
high blood pressure 27, 46, 53, 58, 73, 110
high blood sugar 126
high density lipoproteins 69
high selenium soil 133
histamine allergies 36, 58
Hodgkin's disease 42, 82
hormonal effects upon manganese 118
hormonal imbalance 70
hostility 107
human selenium toxicity 140
hydrochloric acid 147
hydroxyapitite 62
hyper-irritability 67
hyperactive 47, 67
hyperactive children 58
hyperactive reflexes 67
hyperactivity 83, 107, 158
hyperadrenia 42
hypercalcemia 62
hypercalcuria 166
hypercholesterolemia 68, 82, 160, 170
hyperglycemia 36, 73, 83
hyperinsulinism 126
hyperkalemia 150, 166
hypernatremia 150
hyperparathyroid 55
hyperparathyroidism 62
hypertension 41, 42, 50, 68, 83, 143, 150, 151, 153, 160
hyperthyroidism 10, 42, 55, 72, 153, 164
hypertryglyceridemia 68
hypoadrenia 42
hypocalcemia 61
hypochromic anemia 141
hypoglycemia 38, 73, 117, 153
hypokalemia 150
hypoparathyroidism 72

Index

hypotension 42
hypothalamus (Lateral portion) 26
hypothalmus (Medial protion) 26
hypothyroidism 26, 42, 90, 112, 117, 153

I

immune competence 136
immune deficiency 100
immune regulation 70
immune response 136
immune suppression 100
immune system 109
inability to concentrate 67
increased cellular immune response 42
increased humoral immune response 42
increased uric acid 166
indocin 90
infarcts 82
infection 80
Infections (bacterial) 42
Infections (viral) 42
infectious anemia 81, 109
infertility 143
inflammation 30
insecticide dust 163
insecticides 161
insomnia 58, 59, 70, 83
insulin 25, 38, 52, 53, 57, 60, 73, 91, 109, 118, 119, 124, 125, 149
interpretation of TMA 10
intracranial hypertension 108
IQ 158
iron 2, 8, 10, 15, 16, 39, 46, 48, 73, 79, 80, 83, 91, 103, 152, 162
iron and infections 109
iron deficiency 112
iron deficiency anemia 106, 135
iron overload 110
iron requirements 114
iron to copper ratio 79, 81
iron to mercury ratio 162
iron toxicity 110, 121
irregular menses 141
ischemic heart attacks 68
ischemic heart disease 82

J

jaundice 135

K

Kaschin-Beck 4, 134
Keshan disease 4, 134
kidney disease 3, 54, 150, 160
kidney stones 57, 62, 69

L

L-phenylalanine 112
lactation 71
lactic acid 58
laxatives 50, 163

LDL 82, 100
lead 2, 6, 10, 72, 80, 157
lead acetate 6
lead based interior house paints 157
lead contamination in children 157
lead crystal 158
lead line 158
learning disabilities 88, 117, 158
lethargy 86
leukemia 42
leukocytosis 166
leukopenia 141
librium 90
licorice 48
licorice root 48, 111
lipid disorders 70
lipid peroxidation 111
lipoproteins 69
lithium 165
liver 80, 90
liver degeneration 2
liver disease 134
loss of memory 59
loss of smell and taste 100
low blood pressure 28, 37, 61, 153
low body temperature 37
low density lipoproteins 69
low thyroid activity 61
lung cancer 160
lupus 42, 119
lupus erythematosus 97
lymphatic tissues 80
lysyl oxidase 78

M

macular degeneration 100, 143
magnesium 7, 16, 22, 27, 31, 37, 39, 43, 55, 56, 61, 66, 67, 68, 69, 70, 71, 72, 73, 75, 84, 103, 152
magnesium deficiencies 67
malignancies 62, 109
malignancies and copper 82
manganese 4, 46, 48, 73, 117
manganese deficiency 119
manganese toxicity 121
manic depression 100, 165
manic disorders 83
medicated shampoos 7
memory loss 67
Menkes disease 81
menstrual irregularities 99
mental disturbances 4
mental retardation 161
mercury 2, 3, 10, 161
mercury toxicity 106
metabolic activity 35
metabolic individuality 151
metabolic rate 28, 39, 41, 44, 45, 61, 83
metabolic type 10, 11, 34, 41, 50
methionine 166
migraine headaches 50, 110
milk 45
mineral interrelationships 16

mineral synergism 17
minerals antagonistic to calcium 55
minerals antagonistic to chromium 127
minerals antagonistic to copper 92
minerals antagonistic to iron 113
minerals antagonistic to magnesium 72
minerals antagonistic to manganese 120
minerals antagonistic to selenium 138
minerals antagonistic to zinc 101
minerals synergistic to calcium 63
minerals synergistic to chromium 129
minerals synergistic to magnesium 75
minimal brain dysfunction 107
molybdenum 166
molybdenum-copper antagonism 167
monoamine oxidase (MAO) 78, 170
mononucleosis 83
multiple sclerosis 42, 81, 117, 164
muscle cramping 150
muscle cramps 59, 67, 68
muscular complaints 143
muscular contraction 68
muscular dystrophy 143
myelination 81
myocardial infarction 70

N

neomycin 163
neuro-endocrine system 24, 28
neuronal development 107
neuropsychiatric conditions 164
niacin 20, 46
nickel 152, 167
night blindness 21
non-spinal fractures 54
norpramin 90
nutrients synergistic to selenium 139
nutrition 24

O

obesity 129
oral contraceptive agents 26, 84, 98
orinase 90
Osgood Schlaters 119
osteoarthritis 69, 80
osteoblasts 56
osteoclasts 57
osteolytic bone disease 71
osteoporosis 15, 26, 54, 55, 57, 58, 59, 63, 70, 83, 119
ovaries (estrogen) 26
oxalic acid 45, 53
oxidative damage 69
oxytocin 149

P

Paget's disease 62
pagophagia 108
pancreas 25, 39, 52, 73, 91
pancreas (endocrine) 26
pancreatic enzyme 112

pancreatic fibrosis 134
pancreatic hormones 37
pancreatitis 10, 71
panic attacks 59
para-sympathetic 26, 27, 41, 90
para-sympathetic dominance 42
para-sympathetic endocrine 28
para-thyroid 112, 126, 162
paralysis 81
paranoid feelings 59
parasites 163
parathyroid 26, 37, 39, 53, 57, 71, 74, 102
parathyroid gland 39, 56, 57
parathyroid hormone 56, 118
Parkinson's disease 42, 81, 111, 117, 164
pear-shaped 34
peppermint 111
peptic ulcers 36, 100
peripheral neuropathy 125
personality 33
personality traits 36
personality types 41
Perthes disease 119
phenobarbital 53
phosphate 56
phosphorus 10, 16, 22, 27, 28, 37, 39, 52, 54, 55, 57, 62, 103
phytate 71
phytic acid 45, 53, 58
Pica 106, 108
PKU 4, 119
platinum 168
plumbism 158
PMS 42, 45, 84
pneumonitis 160
post menopausal osteoporosis 55
post partum depression 100
post traumatic dysinsulinism 127
post-menstrual syndrome 85, 99
posterior pituitary 26
postpartum depression. 85
postural hypotension 37
potassium 8, 10, 15, 16, 20, 27, 37, 39, 43, 46, 48, 68, 147, 152
pottery 158
pre-eclampsia 70
prednisone 100
pregnancy 28, 79, 80, 85, 100, 126
premature aging 57
premature infants 135
premenstrual syndrome (PMS) 26, 70, 84, 99, 100
pretzels 46
progesterone 26, 84, 85, 99, 149
prolactin 149
prolonged diarrhea 71
prostate 104
prostate enlargement 100
protein 45, 118
protein breakdown 54
protein matrix 54
prunes 45
psoas 62
psoriasis 97

Index

R

recovery stage of stress 28, 29
"relative" deficiency 71
relative zinc deficiency 100
renal disease 71
renin 148
reproductive disorders 160
resistance stage of stress 28, 29
restless legs 62
rheumatoid arthritis 58, 79, 80, 100, 109
rhubarb 45, 53
rickets 8, 21, 50, 160
RNA 67

S

salt craving 149
salt-sensitive 151
schizophrenia 117
scleroderma 97
scoliosis 87
scurvy 93
sedative 48
sedative nutrients 42, 43
seizures 61, 70, 150, 158
selenium 7, 15, 132, 152, 160, 162
selenium deficiency 134, 137
selenium to mercury ratio 162
selenium toxicity 133
senile osteoporosis 54
serum calcium 61
sexual development 96
sickle cell anemia 98
sickle cell disease 4
SIDS 158
signs of acute boron toxicity 163
signs of lead exposure 158
silicon 168
silicosis 169
silver 169
skin conditions 97
slow metabolic type 34, 44, 45, 60, 153
slow metabolism 37, 38, 39, 43, 57
slow wound healing 100
sodium 10, 27, 37, 39, 43, 46, 48, 58, 73, 147
sodium and fluid retention 68
sodium excess 150
sodium retention 152
sodium-insensitive 151
soft water 43, 44
sorghum 45
source of aluminum 162
sources of molybdenum 167
sources of nickel 168
sources of selenium 140, 141
sources of vanadium 170
soy 46
spasticity 81
specific dynamic action 44
spinach 45, 53
spleen 80
sprue 71

staphylococcus aureus 69
steely hair disease 81
sterility 100
stiffness in the joints 57
stimulating nutrients 43
stimulatory 48
stimulatory nutrients 42
stones 69
strenuous exercise 150
stress 27, 28, 33, 36, 37, 66, 70, 71, 72, 126, 153
stress glands 27
stress induced heart attack 68
stress-aholics 35
stretch marks 97
strontium 169
stunted growth 96
sudden infant death syndrome (SIDS) 136
sulfur 137, 160, 162, 166, 169
sulfur to mercury ratio 162
superoxide dismutase 78, 118
superoxide radicals 118
sympathetic 26, 27, 28, 39, 41
sympathetic and parasympathetic nervous system 24
sympathetic dominance 42, 43
sympathetic endocrines 27, 90
sympathetic nervous 149
symptoms of acute arsenic toxicity 160
symptoms of chronic arsenic toxicity 160
symptoms of cobalt deficiency 163
symptoms of cobalt toxicity 164
symptoms of gold toxicity 165
symptoms of mercury toxicity 161
symptoms of selenium toxicity 140
synergistic nutrients 103
synergistic relationship 15
synergistic vitamins to iron 114
systolic hypertension 68

T

tannin 119
tapazol 90
tardive dyskinesia 121
tegretol 90
tendinitis 62
tetany 61, 70
thiamin 46, 74
thiocyanates 45
thorazine 90
thyroid 25, 35, 37, 39, 56, 57, 60, 71, 82, 102, 108, 118, 126, 137
thyroid gland 53, 57
thyroid insufficiency 90
thyroxine 112
tin 170
tissue calcium 61
tissue mineral analysis 2
tissue mineral analysis (TMA) and zinc analysis 103
titanium 170
TMA 2, 9, 10
toxemia 85
toxic heavy metals 2
toxic metals 28, 72, 156

toxic shock syndrome 69
tremors 81
triglyceride 82
TSH 165
tumor growth 82
type A personality 33, 35, 152
type B personality 33
type I osteoporosis 56
type II insomnia 37
type II osteoporosis 57
tyramine 50
tyrosinase 78

U

ulcers (gastric) 42
ulcers (peptic or duodenal) 42

V

vanadium 170
vegetarians 38, 83, 100
very low density lipoproteins 69
viral 28
viral infection 38, 60, 83, 86, 93
viruses 22, 60, 99, 100, 153
vitamin A 8, 18, 21, 22, 56, 87, 99, 103
vitamin B1 74, 103
vitamin B12 42, 75, 114
vitamin B2 163
vitamin B3 103
vitamin B5 103
vitamin B6 69, 74, 84, 100, 103
vitamin C 8, 15, 16, 20, 21, 22, 56, 62, 74, 87, 93
vitamin D 8, 16, 20, 21, 22, 42, 50, 53, 54, 55, 56, 57, 59, 62, 74, 114, 160, 163
vitamin E 18, 22, 42, 74, 75, 102, 103, 114, 132, 135, 136, 160
vitamin interrelationships 18
vitamin needs 7
vitamin synergists 19
vitamin-mineral interrelationships 20
vitamin-mineral synergism 21, 62, 75
vitamins antagonistic to calcium 56
vitamins antagonistic to copper 92
vitamins antagonistic to iron 113
vitamins antagonistic to magnesium 74
vitamins antagonistic to manganese 120
vitamins antagonistic to selenium 139
vitamins antagonistic to zinc 102
vitamins synergistic to calcium 63
vitamins synergistic to chromium 129
vitamins synergistic to magnesium 75

W

water 43, 110
water balance 149
weight gain 84, 99
weightlessness 55
white muscle disease 132
Wilson's disease 2, 83

X

xanthine oxidase 166
xenobiotics 135

Y

yeast 87
yeast infections 42

Z

zinc 8, 10, 16, 21, 39, 55, 57, 80, 83, 84, 87, 96, 136, 162
zinc deficiency 96, 100
zinc overload 100
zinc requirements 103
zinc/copper antagonism 91
zinc/copper ratio 88, 89, 99
zinc/mercury ratio 162
zirconium 171